Arthritis and Rheumatism

IN PRACTICE

Arthritis and Rheumatism

IN PRACTICE

Paul Dieppe
BSc MD FRCP

ARC Professor of Rheumatology
Bristol Royal Infirmary
Bristol, UK

Cyrus Cooper
MA DM MRCP

Senior Registrar
Bristol Royal Infirmary
Bristol, UK

John Kirwan
BSc MD MRCP

Consultant Senior Lecturer
in Rheumatology
Bristol Royal Infirmary
Bristol, UK

Neil McGill
MB BS BSc (Med)
FRACP

Consultant Rheumatologist
Royal Prince Alfred and
Rachel Forster Hospitals,
Sydney, Australia

Advisors:

John Dickson
MB ChB MRCGP FRCP

General Practitioner, Northallerton, UK
Chairman, Primary Care
Rheumatology Society, UK

Roger Atkins
MA MB BS FRCS DM

Consultant Senior Lecturer in
Orthopaedic Surgery, Bristol Royal
Infirmary, UK

Gower Medical Publishing LONDON • NEW YORK
J.B. Lippincott Company PHILADELPHIA

Distributed in USA and Canada by:
J.B. Lippincott Company
East Washington Square
Philadelphia, PA 19105
USA

Gower Medical Publishing
101 Fifth Avenue
New York, NY 10003
USA

Distributed in UK, Europe and rest of world by:
Gower Medical Publishing
Middlesex House
34–42 Cleveland Street
London W1P 5FB
UK

Distributed in Japan by:
Igaku Shoin Ltd
Tokyo International
P.O. Box 5063
Tokyo
Japan

Publisher: Fiona Foley

Project editor: Alison Whitehouse

Designer: Erminia Bocchio

Line artist: Marion Tasker

Production: Susan Bishop

Index: J. Roderick Gibb

British Library Cataloguing in Publication Data:
Arthritis and rheumatism in practice.
1. Man. Joints. Arthritis & rheumatic diseases
I. Dieppe, P.A. (Paul Adrian)
616.72

Library of Congress Cataloging-in-Publication Data:
Arthritis and rheumatism in practice
Paul Dieppe ... [et al.]; advisors. John Dickson.
    Roger Atkins.
Includes index.
1. Arthritis.   2. Rheumatism.   I. Dieppe, Paul.
[DNLM: 1. Arthritis.   2. Pain.   3. Rheumatic Diseases
WE 344 A78703]
RC933.A6618   1990
616.7′22--dc20

ISBN: 0 397 44588 1 (Lippincott/Gower)

Typesetting by M to N Typesetters, London

Text set in Rotation Roman; captions set in Rotation Italic;
figures set in Optima Light Condensed

Originated in Hong Kong by Bright Arts
Printed in Singapore 1990 by Imago Producions (FE) Pte Ltd
Print No. 5,4,3,2,1

PREFACE

Musculoskeletal disorders are a common and important cause of ill health. Although rheumatology is an expanding subspecialty of general medicine, hospital-based rheumatologists can only see a minority of patients with these disorders, leaving the great majority to be treated by their primary care physician.

Most current textbooks of rheumatology are written by specialists, for specialists. Even those written for the student or general practitioner are often biased towards hospital-based practice, including, for example, lengthy sections on uncommon diseases. The publishers and authors of this book perceived the need for a relatively small, user-friendly book aimed specifically at providing information about the common conditions seen in the community. In order to achieve this, and to bridge the gap between rheumatologists and primary care physicians, we have sought the advice of colleagues in general practice and placed emphasis on common problems as they might present in the surgery.

We are particularly grateful to Mr Roger Atkins and Dr John Dickson. Both have advised us on the contents of the book from the outset, and made helpful suggestions on the whole manuscript. We would also like to thank Alison Whitehouse and her colleagues at Gower Medical Publishing for excellent support and advice, and Erminia Bocchio for the superb design and artwork.

PAD, CC, JRK, NWMcG
Bristol, July 1990

CONTENTS

Section 1

INTRODUCTION

INTRODUCTION

Arthritis and Rheumatism in Practice is an aid to diagnosis and management of common musculoskeletal problems which present in every surgery. We have written it from the perspective of hospital rheumatology but with advice from an orthopaedic surgeon and a general practitioner with a special interest in arthritis and rheumatism.

About one in twenty of the under-40s and one in three of the over-60s suffer from arthritis and rheumatism. Some 80% of those who suffer do nothing about it, the other 20% go to a primary care physician, and less than 1% are referred to a hospital. The number seeking help is rising as the population becomes generally older and fitter, and as our tolerance of symptoms and disability becomes less. Clearly *Arthritis and Rheumatism in Practice* needs to be about practical issues in diagnosis and management of the common rheumatic problems seen in the community (Fig. 1). Hospital-based concepts of rheumatology are often of little relevance to the vast majority of sufferers, carers and doctors. We therefore aim to provide a synopsis of the major musculoskeletal disorders affecting the general population, and a concise approach to their management.

The basic structure of the book is shown in Figures 2 and 3. We open with a brief review of the pathological processes that result in musculoskeletal disease. Rheumatology is a young specialty, and advances in our understanding of common disorders have emerged in the relatively recent past. In the section on approaches to pathology and diagnosis, this pathological basis is translated to the clinical classification of rheumatic disease. The emphasis here is on the principles, rather than the detail, of specific processes, and we hope to link these processes with clinical outcomes.

The main section covers the most frequent regional presentations of musculoskeletal disorders. In these, we consistently address the functional anatomy, physical examination, investigation and management of the commoner conditions. For each regional site, a detailed analysis is given of the most common disorders in general practice. This is accompanied by a subsection ('Not to be Missed') in which groups of conditions are listed which are less frequent but have more sinister implications if missed. Specific aspects of the management of the commoner disorders are also discussed in this section, for ease of reference.

We conclude by concisely highlighting the major facets of management of rheumatic disorders. Drug therapy, though important among these, must be integrated into a general approach with education, exercise, and the provision of aids and appliances. One of our aims here is to provide some concrete examples of how these general approaches can be applied to the needs of individual patients, and we have therefore included a series of relevant case histories.

We hope that this volume will serve more as a practical manual than a rheumatology textbook. We have concentrated on common problems at the expense of 'small print', and have been didactic on occasion in our examination and management

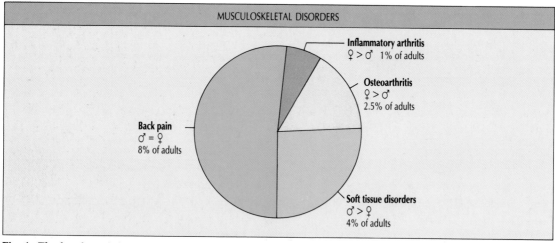

Fig. 1 *The burden of rheumatic diseases on the community.*

strategies. The standard format and colour-coded pages are intended to enable rapid reference in the consulting room or on the practice bookshelf, while the illustrations and tables aim to convey the important aspects of rheumatology in a concise fashion.

As with the specialty itself, the art of teaching rheumatology is young. We feel that this volume represents a departure from the format of most short textbooks currently available, and hope that it will provide a rational, yet practical, framework for coping with the burden of arthritis and rheumatism in practice.

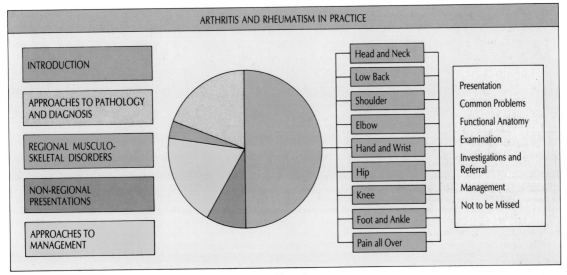

Fig. 2 *The structure of* Arthritis and Rheumatism in Practice.

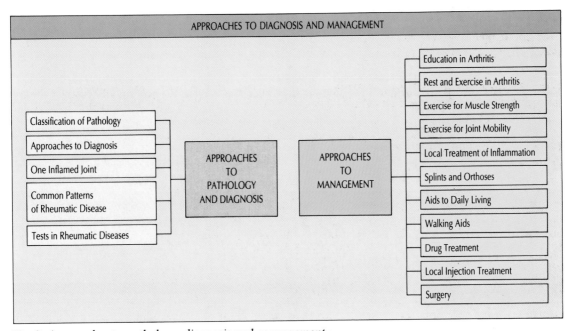

Fig. 3 *Approaches to pathology, diagnosis and management.*

Section 2

APPROACHES TO PATHOLOGY AND DIAGNOSIS

CLASSIFICATION OF PATHOLOGY

The basic structure of a synovial joint is shown in Figure 1. Pathological processes may be categorized into three groups according to the structures involved: (i) articular, (ii) periarticular, and (iii) referred.

Articular

The joint itself comprises the bone ends, articular cartilage, synovium and joint capsule. Joint disorders are of two main types (Fig. 2):

- **Inflammatory arthritis,** for example rheumatoid arthritis, is dominated by inflammation in the synovium which is followed by damage to articular cartilage and subchondral bone.

- **Osteoarthritis and related disorders** are characterized by focal cartilage loss with subchondral bone reaction and only mild synovitis.

Typical clinical features of all articular disorders include pain that is worse on movement, joint tenderness that can be elicited all the way round the joint margin, and painful restriction of passive joint movement. In addition, there may be signs of inflammation (warmth, effusion) or crepitus.

Periarticular

Soft tissue periarticular disorders fall into two broad groups:

- **Synovial:** involving the synovial lining of bursae and tendon sheaths. These disorders are most often a result of repetitive trauma or inflammatory synovial disorders such as rheumatoid arthritis.

- **Insertional:** involving the insertions of tendons and ligaments into bone (Fig. 3). These are most often caused by severe trauma or by certain inflammatory joint disorders such as ankylosing spondylitis.

Referred

Joint pain may be referred in three ways:

- **Nerves** (and their roots) may be irritated at their exit foramina from the vertebral column or during their subsequent course, giving rise to symptoms and signs distally.

- **Local referral of pain** (or tenderness), for example

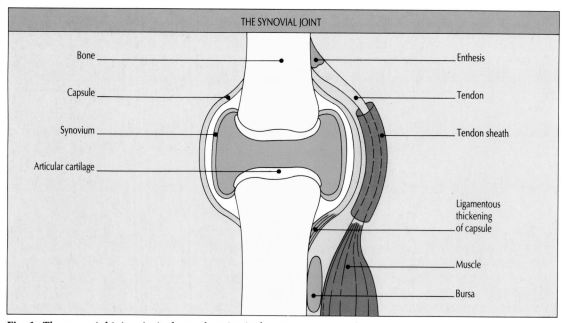

Fig. 1 *The synovial joint. Articular and periarticular structures are shown.*

pain in the knee or muscles of the thigh resulting from arthritis of the apophyseal joints in the lumbar spine.

- **Visceral structures** may cause poorly localized pain in other sites, for example shoulder pain in ischaemic heart disease.

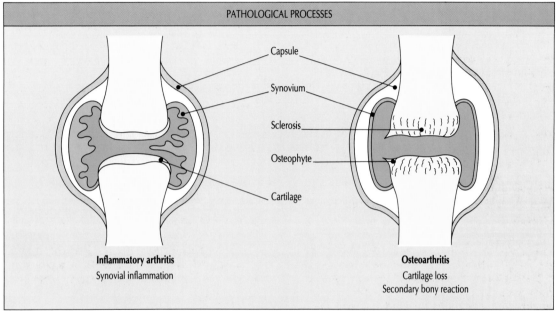

Fig. 2 *Pathological processes in inflammatory arthritis (left) and osteoarthritis (right).*

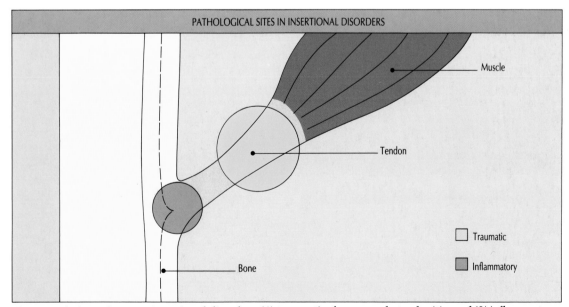

Fig. 3 *Pathological sites in insertional disorders: (1) traumatic, for example tendonitis, and (2) inflammatory, for example ankylosing spondylitis.*

APPROACHES TO DIAGNOSIS

How to .... tell if a patient has nerve root pain

This is difficult and can be confused with radiating pain from various spinal sites. Check for:

Symptoms in the spine ⟶
- local pain and stiffness
- asymmetrical paraspinal muscle spasm.

Radiation of symptoms ⟶
- sharp pain in characteristic distribution
- dermatomal sensory change (hyperaesthesia, anaesthesia, paraesthesia)
- motor weakness in appropriate muscles.

Reflexes ⟶
- diminished or lost reflex.

Nerve irritation ⟶
- on moving the spine (e.g. turning head) *or*
- on moving the nerve (e.g. straight leg raising) increases *peripheral symptoms.*

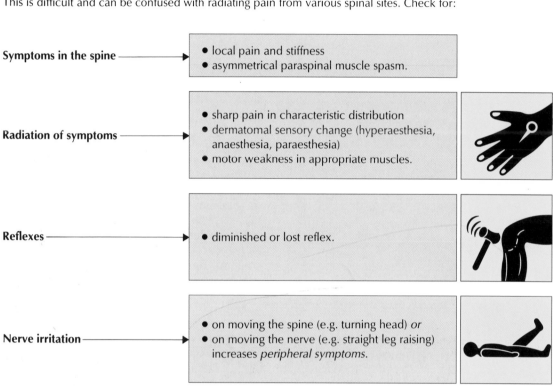

More signs = more certainty

THINGS WHICH GO TOGETHER			
Sensory change	*Motor weakness*	*Reflexes*	*Nerve root*
Deltoid region	Shoulder abduction	Biceps	C5
Thumb & index finger	Wrist extension	Supinator	C6
Middle finger	Elbow extension	Triceps	C7
Little & ring fingers	Finger flexion	–	C8
Ulnar aspect forearm	Small hand muscles	–	T1
Front of thigh	Hip flexion & adduction	–	L2
Front of knee	Knee extension	Knee	L3
Inner shin	Ankle dorsiflexion	(knee)	L4
Outer shin; dorsum of foot	Big toe dorsiflexion	–	L5
Outer border of foot; sole	Knee flexion; foot plantar flexion	Ankle	S1

Note: Local tenderness often occurs in areas of dermatomal symptom radiation.

How to .... tell if a patient has peripheral nerve entrapment

Ask about characteristic symptoms ——→
- shooting pain
- pain radiating distally
- often worse at night.

Check for characteristic signs ——→
- usually sensory loss
- may have hyperaesthesia
- does not fit a nerve root distribution.

Sensory loss is common ——→
- in median nerve compression at the wrist (carpal tunnel syndrome)

- in ulnar nerve entrapment at the elbow.

How to .... tell if a patient has tendonitis

Tendon inflammation may occur ——→
- at the site of tendon insertion
- along the tendon's course
- within tendon sheaths.

Inflamed tendons are ——→
- tender to pressure
- painful when actively used against resistance
- usually painless on passive movement
- unlikely to restrict joint movement.

Common Sites of Tendonitis ——→

supraspinatus

triceps

biceps

Achilles

de Quervain's

How to ....
.... assess the activity of inflammatory arthritis

The inflammatory activity of arthritis is best assessed by asking about the symptoms of pain and stiffness, counting the number of inflamed joints, checking the acute phase response and looking for new joint damage.

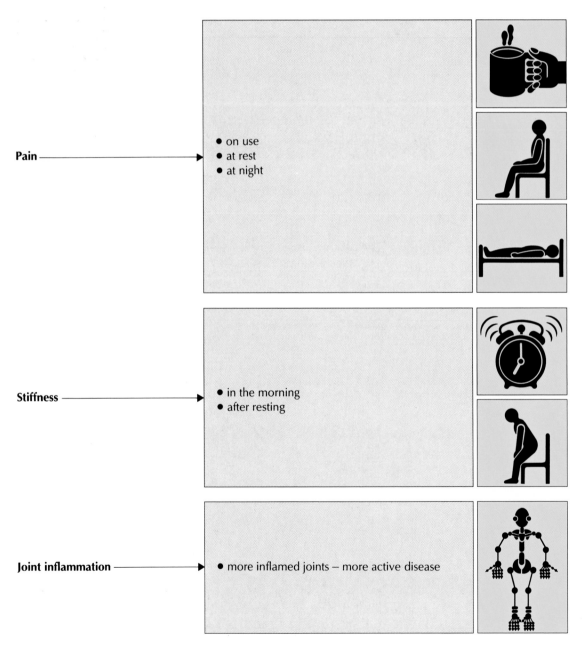

Pain
- on use
- at rest
- at night

Stiffness
- in the morning
- after resting

Joint inflammation
- more inflamed joints – more active disease

Investigations ──────▶

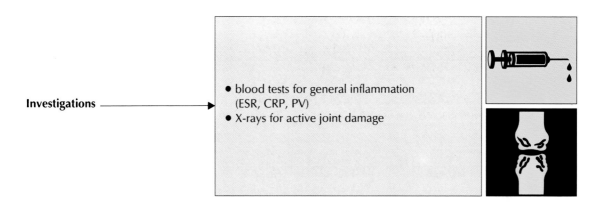

- blood tests for general inflammation (ESR, CRP, PV)
- X-rays for active joint damage

How to ....
.... tell if a patient has bursitis

Inflammation of bursae produces ──────▶

- tenderness on, but not nearby, the bursa, which can be identified with a single finger
- local swelling if the bursa is near the surface
- pain on stretching the tissues (ligaments or tendons) over the bursa
- a diffuse ache near the bursa.

Bursitis does not usually cause pain on moving nearby joints passively.

Common sites of bursitis ──────▶

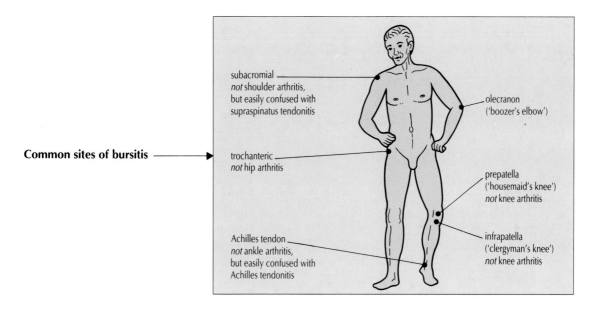

subacromial
not shoulder arthritis, but easily confused with supraspinatus tendonitis

olecranon ('boozer's elbow')

trochanteric
not hip arthritis

prepatella ('housemaid's knee')
not knee arthritis

Achilles tendon
not ankle arthritis, but easily confused with Achilles tendonitis

infrapatella ('clergyman's knee')
not knee arthritis

2.7

How to ....
.... assess functional loss

Functional loss may be related to specific regions: the hands, shoulders and legs are the most common ones. The overall functional status of the patient can be summarized with reference to important everyday activities.

Specific regions

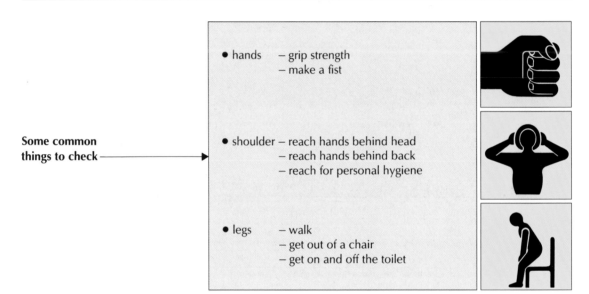

Some common
things to check

- hands — grip strength
  — make a fist

- shoulder — reach hands behind head
  — reach hands behind back
  — reach for personal hygiene

- legs — walk
  — get out of a chair
  — get on and off the toilet

General function

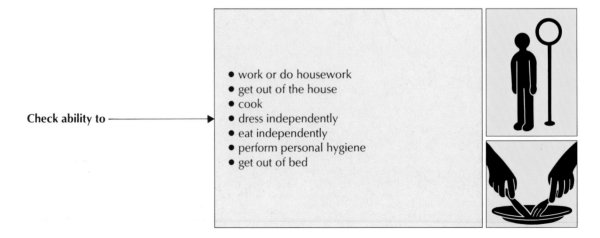

Check ability to

- work or do housework
- get out of the house
- cook
- dress independently
- eat independently
- perform personal hygiene
- get out of bed

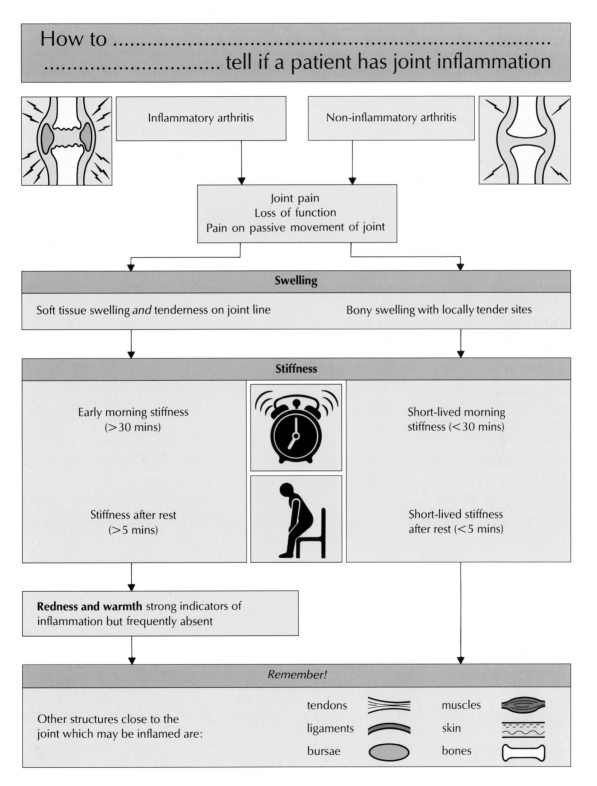

How to ....
.... tell if a patient has joint inflammation

Inflammatory arthritis

Non-inflammatory arthritis

Joint pain
Loss of function
Pain on passive movement of joint

Swelling

Soft tissue swelling *and* tenderness on joint line

Bony swelling with locally tender sites

Stiffness

Early morning stiffness
(>30 mins)

Short-lived morning
stiffness (<30 mins)

Stiffness after rest
(>5 mins)

Short-lived stiffness
after rest (<5 mins)

Redness and warmth strong indicators of
inflammation but frequently absent

Remember!

Other structures close to the
joint which may be inflamed are:

tendons	muscles
ligaments	skin
bursae	bones

Presentation

An acutely painful joint developing over 24–48 hours presents the threat of potentially rapid joint destruction and provides the opportunity of an accurate and specific diagnosis – it is thus essential that appropriate investigation be instituted without delay. Recurrent bouts of acute arthritis that have settled spontaneously, or with non-steroidal anti-inflammatory drug therapy, suggest a crystal induced arthritis, or, less commonly, an inflammatory arthritis such as palindromic rheumatism. Subacute arthritis of one joint suggests an inflammatory arthritis such as rheumatoid or an unusual infection.

Examination

Check the painful joint to differentiate arthritis from periarthritis, then search for minor involvement of other joints and for a source of infection.

LOOK: for external signs. A hot, shiny, red, swollen joint, as shown in Figure 1, is almost always the site of sepsis or crystal-induced inflammation. The presence of fever and other constitutional symptoms, when only one joint is involved, strongly suggest sepsis. Trauma, sufficient to produce an acutely swollen painful knee, will usually bruise or otherwise mark the skin.

FEEL: for warmth and tenderness, which are most notable in septic and (pseudo)gouty joints. Osteomyelitis may lead to the occurrence of a joint (sympathetic) effusion but maximal tenderness will usually be located away from the joint line.

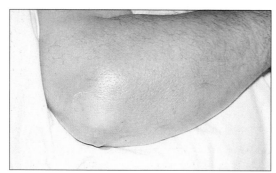

Fig. 1 *Septic arthritis of the elbow joint showing swelling with overlying oedema and redness.*

MOVE: the joint. Acutely inflamed (especially septic and gouty) joints are very painful to move.

Common Problems

Common causes of an acutely painful joint include:

- **Trauma:** major trauma is usually obvious as the cause of acute pain in and around a joint. Beware of accepting minor trauma as the cause of an acutely swollen joint, especially when there is a delay between the episode of trauma and the onset of symptoms: in this situation it is best to actively exclude other possibilities. Management of trauma is discussed in relation to specific joint sites in the other sections.

- **Gout and pseudogout:** the easiest time to obtain definitive proof of these diagnoses is when the patient presents with an acutely swollen joint. This opportunity for joint aspiration and synovial fluid examination should not be missed (see 'Management', below).

- **Haemarthrosis:** contamination of synovial fluid with blood at the time of aspiration is relatively common and should be differentiated from uniformly blood stained fluid or frank haemarthrosis, which are indicative of intra-articular bleeding. Most cases of haemarthrosis are due to trauma; less commonly the cause is haemophilia, pseudogout or sepsis.

- **Inflammatory arthritides:** such as rheumatoid or psoriatic arthritis or Reiter's disease, usually involve several joints but may affect only one joint.

Not to be Missed

- **Sepsis.** By far the most important diagnosis to be considered in the patient with an acutely inflamed joint is sepsis – undiagnosed or undertreated it will produce rapid joint destruction (Fig. 2). Chronic destructive arthritis, drug addiction and sexual promiscuity (gonococcus) all increase the risk. An associated tenosynovitis increases the likelihood of a gonococcal etiology (Fig. 3).

  Thorough investigation *before* antibiotics are given is essential; this is best handled in a hospital emergency department. Cultures of synovial fluid, blood and other sites (especially for gonococcus) should be obtained. Treatment should commence with intravenous antibiotics, selected with the help of the Gram-stain findings and subsequently by the antibiotic sensitivities of the culture. Repeat aspiration or surgical drainage may be required.

  Septic arthritis requires intensive and prolonged therapy, usually for 4–12 weeks. After antibiotic treatment has started and the joint has begun to settle, physiotherapy to regain mobility and function should commence.

Investigations and Referral

The key investigation for acute arthritis is aspiration of the inflamed joint (Figs 4 & 5). The synovial fluid obtained should be examined for organisms by

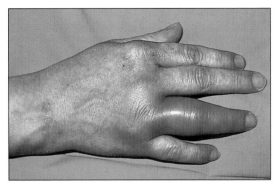

Fig. 3 *Gonococcal tenosynovitis in a 24-year-old woman. Courtesy of Dr S.E. Thompson.*

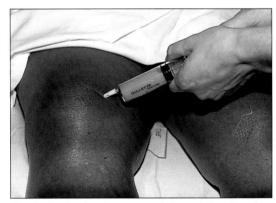

Fig. 4 *Aspiration from a septic knee joint. A wide-bore needle is used to obtain the thick exudate.*

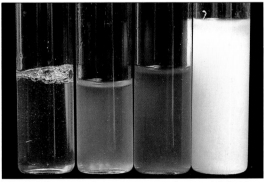

Fig. 5 *Macroscopic appearance of synovial fluids. From left to right: normal (viscous and clear); mild synovial inflammation; mild synovial inflammation with blood-staining due to trauma; severe synovial inflammation (thin and opaque due to very high polymorph count).*

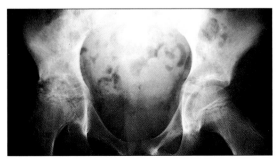

Fig. 2 *Radiograph of a child's hip showing destruction due to sepsis of only 2 weeks' duration.*

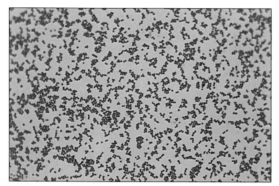

Fig. 6 *Gram-positive cocci in synovial fluid, later confirmed to be* Staphylococcus aureus *on culture. Courtesy of Dr D. Seal.*

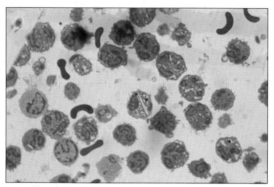

Fig. 7 *Synovial fluid phagocytosis of urate crystals in a uridine-stained sectioned cell pellet (urate crystals under polarized light are shown in 'Tests in Rheumatic Disease', Fig. 7).*

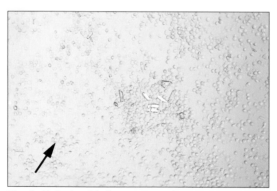

Fig. 8 *Polarized light micrograph of pyrophosphate crystals in blood-stained synovial fluid illustrating the positive sign of birefringence. First order red compensator (arrow).*

Gram-stain and culture (Fig. 6), and by polarized light microscopy for the presence of crystals (Figs 7 & 8). Aspiration should be performed without delay and always prior to the introduction of antibiotics. Gout and pseudogout may both be precipitated by septic arthritis; so even when crystals are seen in the synovial fluid, the joint may still be infected.

A raised white cell count is suggestive of sepsis, but an elevated ESR can be expected in most of the conditions mentioned above and is thus of little diagnostic help. X-Ray of an acute joint usually shows only soft tissue swelling, but the finding of chondrocalcinosis (Fig. 9) or fracture may be diagnostic.

If sepsis is suspected then urgent referral to hospital is indicated.

Management

Gout

Attacks of gout occur when the inflammatory system interacts with intra-articular deposits of monosodium urate crystals. A history of recurrent, abrupt-onset attacks of acute arthritis affecting the first metatarso-phalangeal joint (Fig. 10) is classical, but less typical presentations (Fig. 11) are also common. Other diseases can mimic gout very closely, so it is worthwhile confirming the diagnosis by aspiration of an involved joint at least once for each patient. Treatment of the acute attack consists of rest and a non-steroidal anti-inflammatory drug (for example indomethacin 50 mg, three times daily) in full, but not supranormal, doses until the attack has settled. If non-steroidal anti-inflammatory drug therapy is contraindicated, then medium-dose colchicine (0.5 mg, two tablets twice daily, reduced if diarrhoea occurs), intra-articular steroid or intramuscular depot tetracosactrin (synthetic adrenocorticotrophic hormone, 1 mg) may be used. Allopurinol and other hypouricaemic drugs should not be commenced during an attack of gout (see below), as they will serve to perpetuate, not resolve, the attack.

Long-term hypouricaemic therapy is indicated when there is evidence of joint damage (erosions on X-ray), tophi, renal calculi, chronic gouty inflammation or frequent acute attacks. Hypouricaemic therapy needs to be life-long and there is rarely any need to start urgently – much better that the diagnosis be certain (urate crystals identified in synovial fluid or tophus) and the patient fully understand the necessity for prolonged treatment.

Allopurinol should be commenced after any acute gout has settled and the dose adjusted to bring the serum uric acid level below 0.40 mmol/l. The dose should not usually exceed 400 mg/day, and much lower doses must be used in the present of renal insufficiency. Low-dose colchicine prophylaxis (0.5 mg, one tablet twice daily for 6 months) will prevent the increase in attacks of acute gout which otherwise follow the introduction of hypouricaemic therapy. Uricosuric drugs (probenecid, sulphinpyrazone) may also be used either instead of, or in addition to, allopurinol, provided there is no history of renal calculi and renal function is adequate (glomerular filtration rate > 50 ml/min).

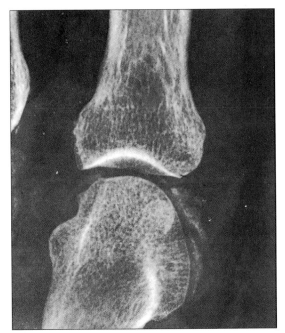 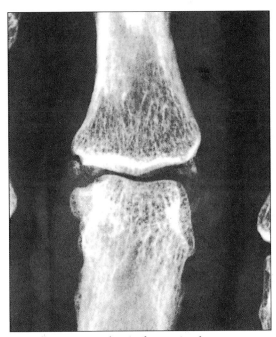

Fig. 9 *Chondrocalcinosis in a patient who developed acute inflammation of a single proximal interphalangeal joint: metacarpophalangeal joint (left); and proximal interphalangeal joint (right). Pyrophosphate crystals were found in the synovial fluid.*

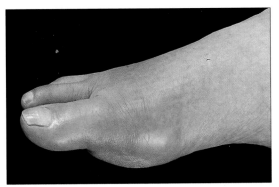 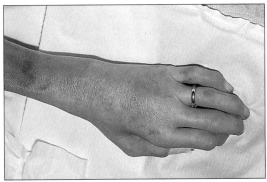

Fig. 10 *The swollen, red, shiny appearance of the toe in early acute gout.*

Fig. 11 *A polyarticular attack of gout affecting the wrist and fingers.*

COMMON PATTERNS OF RHEUMATIC DISEASE

Only a few of the 200 or so different rheumatic diseases occur commonly. The diagnoses can usually be made clinically; investigations are often unnecessary and can be misleading (see 'Tests in Rheumatic Diseases').

Pattern Recognition

There are four main components to clinical pattern recognition:

- **The age, sex, race, and sometimes the family history,** of the patient will determine what is most likely.
- **The mode of onset** (acute or chronic) and chronology of the disorder reflect the pathology.
- **The distribution of involved joints** – both anatomically and in time of involvement – is often characteristic of a specific disease.
- **Associated features in other systems** (the skin, eyes or genital tract for example) may provide further clues to the diagnosis.

Likely Diagnoses by Age and Sex

Most of the common rheumatic diseases have a predilection for persons of a certain age, sex or race (Fig. 1). Gout, for example, rarely affects premenopausal women; ankylosing spondylitis occurs mainly in men, usually starting in their twenties; and polymyalgia rheumatica hardly ever occurs below the age of 60.

Some Common Patterns of Rheumatic Disease

RHEUMATOID ARTHRITIS (RA): A common disease with a peak onset in the 30s and 40s; women are affected three times as frequently as men. The onset is very variable, but often insidious, involving peripheral joints first (hands, wrists and metatarsophalangeal joints), with malaise and marked morning stiffness. Joint disease usually becomes symmetrical and the distribution in the hand is characteristic (Figs 2 & 3). Tests may be misleading in the early stages (see 'Tests in Rheumatic Diseases').

RHEUMATIC DISORDERS AT DIFFERENT AGES			
	Age	Females	Males
Children	0–16 years	Trauma, post-viral, irritable hip (Juvenile chronic arthritis)	
Young adults	17–35 years	Rheumatoid arthritis (Systemic lupus erythematosus) (Psoriatic arthritis)	Reactive arthritis Ankylosing spondylitis (Rheumatoid arthritis)
Middle-aged	36–65 years	Rheumatoid arthritis Osteoarthritis	Gout Rheumatoid arthritis
Elderly	>65 years	Osteoarthritis Rheumatoid arthritis Polymyalgia rheumatica Gout and pseudogout	

Fig. 1 *A simple guide to likely rheumatic disorders at different ages in men and women. (Only the more common diseases are noted; those in parentheses are a little less prevalent than the others.)*

OSTEOARTHRITIS (OA): By far the commonest rheumatic disease, OA has a peak onset in middle age and affects women more often than men. Onset is usually insidious with the gradual development of use-related pain and stiffness. The common joint sites are the knee, hand, hip and spine. Men are more likely to have a single joint affected; women often have a combination of knee and hand disease, with a characteristic pattern of joint involvement (Figs 3 & 4).

GOUT: A common disorder of middle-aged men, although it may be over-diagnosed. Elderly women on diuretics can also develop the disease. Acute attacks often affect the base of the big toe, with the hindfoot or hand joints the next most frequent sites. Most, but not all, attacks are monoarticular. Obesity, hypertension, hyperlipidaemia, cardio-vascular disease and a high beer intake are frequent

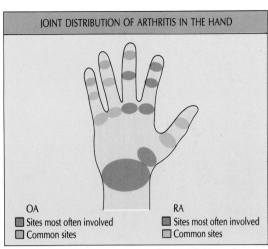

Fig. 3 *Distribution of osteoarthritis (OA) and rheumatoid arthritis (RA) in the hand. Note the inverse distribution of the two diseases.*

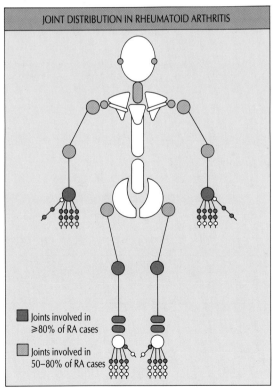

Fig. 2 *Distribution of joint involvement in rheumatoid arthritis. Note the symmetry as well as the characteristic distribution in the hands and feet.*

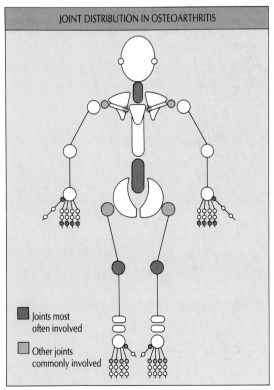

Fig. 4 *Distribution of joints involved in OA. Almost any joint can be involved in elderly people or due to major trauma. The most common combination is knee, hand and spine disease in middle-aged women.*

associations. Typical attacks are excruciatingly painful with red shiny skin over the affected joint (Figs 5 & 6). Serum uric acid levels may be misleading.

PSEUDOGOUT: Is a common cause of acute arthritis in the elderly, usually affecting the knee (Figs 7 & 8) which is less vicious than gout but is likewise caused by crystals (calcium pyrophosphate dihydrate).

ANKYLOSING SPONDYLITIS (AS): Affects men about three times more often than women, and peaks in early adults. Onset is usually insidious with back pain, radiating to the buttocks or legs, that may be mistaken for sciatica (Fig. 9). There is morning stiffness and the pain may be relieved by exercise. A family history is common and iritis may occur.

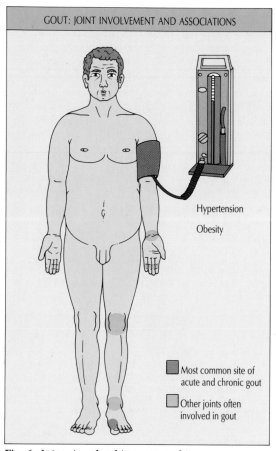

GOUT: JOINT INVOLVEMENT AND ASSOCIATIONS

Hypertension

Obesity

■ Most common site of acute and chronic gout

□ Other joints often involved in gout

Fig. 6 *Joints involved in gout, and its common associations.*

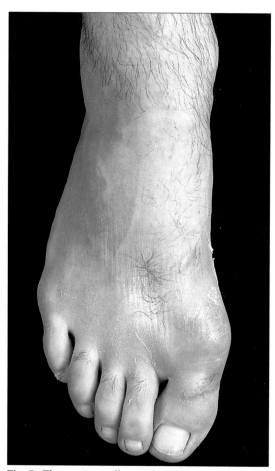

Fig. 5 *The toe is swollen, red and shiny in early acute gout.*

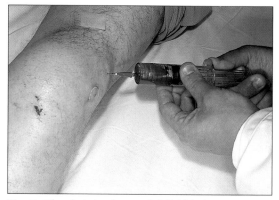

Fig. 7 *Blood-stained synovial fluid being withdrawn from an acutely inflamed knee joint in an attack of pseudogout exacerbated by minor trauma.*

REACTIVE ARTHRITIS: A relatively common disorder in young adults, affecting men more than women. The arthritis is usually in the lower limbs and asymmetrical (Fig. 10). Some or all of the commonly associated features are usually present; these include conjunctivitis, urethritis or cervicitis, mouth ulcers and a pustular rash on the feet (keratoderma blenorrhagica). There is often a history of a nonspecific urethritis or a diarrhoeal illness preceding the disease by 1–4 weeks. (The classical 'Reiter's' triad of conjunctivitis, urethritis and arthritis sometimes occurs.)

PSORIATIC ARTHRITIS: Some 10% of people with psoriasis develop arthritis. This can take a number of forms, including disorders that are very similar to AS or RA. In addition, 'sausage-like' swellings of a finger or toe, or arthritis of the distal

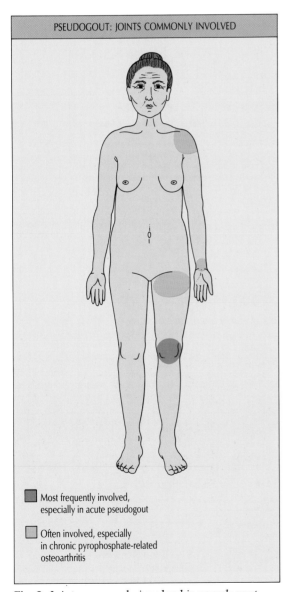

PSEUDOGOUT: JOINTS COMMONLY INVOLVED

■ Most frequently involved, especially in acute pseudogout

■ Often involved, especially in chronic pyrophosphate-related osteoarthritis

Fig. 8 *Joints commonly involved in pseudogout.*

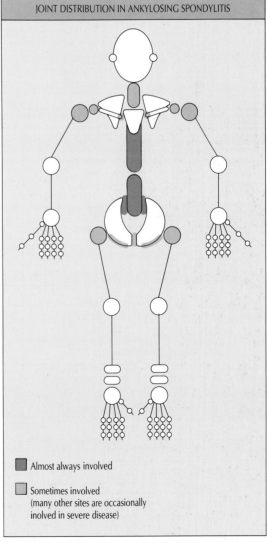

JOINT DISTRIBUTION IN ANKYLOSING SPONDYLITIS

■ Almost always involved

■ Sometimes involved (many other sites are occasionally involved in severe disease)

Fig. 9 *Distribution of joint involvement in ankylosing spondylitis. Note the symmetry and the central distribution.*

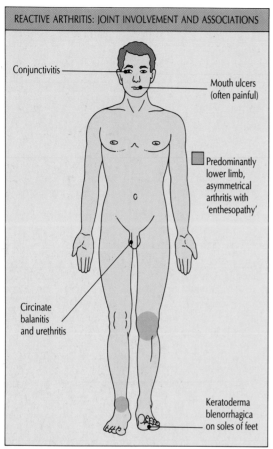

REACTIVE ARTHRITIS: JOINT INVOLVEMENT AND ASSOCIATIONS

Conjunctivitis

Mouth ulcers
(often painful)

Predominantly
lower limb,
asymmetrical
arthritis with
'enthesopathy'

Circinate
balanitis
and urethritis

Keratoderma
blenorrhagica
on soles of feet

Fig. 10 *Joints involved in reactive arthritis, and its common associations. The lower limb is affected, predominantly, with asymmetrical arthritis with 'enthesopathy'.*

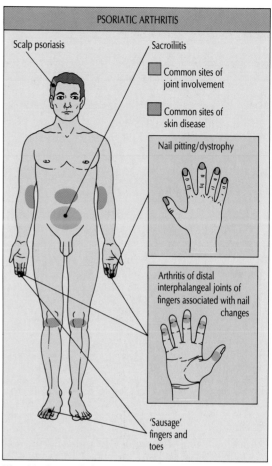

PSORIATIC ARTHRITIS

Scalp psoriasis

Sacroiliitis

Common sites of
joint involvement

Common sites of
skin disease

Nail pitting/dystrophy

Arthritis of distal
interphalangeal joints of
fingers associated with nail
changes

'Sausage'
fingers and
toes

Fig. 11 *Sites of skin and joint lesions in psoriatic arthritis (a symmetrical polyarthritis can also occur).*

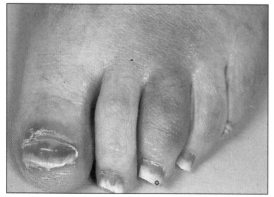

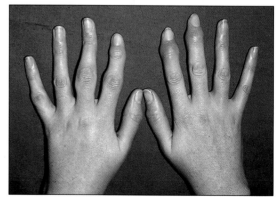

Fig. 12 *Psoriatic arthritis. 'Sausage-like' swelling (left) and distal interphalangeal joint arthritis (right) occur in the hands and feet.*

interphalangeal joints, may develop (Figs 11 & 12). The disorder is very variable.

CONNECTIVE TISSUE DISORDERS: An odd group of uncommon, multi-system disorders principally affecting young women, associated with immuno-logical abnormalities. Systemic lupus erythematosus is the commonest, and affects black and Oriental women more than Caucasians. Suspicious features include malaise, depression, skin rashes, hair loss and mouth ulcers, in addition to joint pains (Fig. 13). A wide variety of presentations and complications can occur.

POLYMYALGIA RHEUMATICA: A relatively common disorder of elderly men and women. The onset may be acute or chronic. The condition is characterized by pain and stiffness of the shoulder and pelvic girdles, much worse in the morning (patients frequently say they cannot get out of bed) (Fig. 14). Malaise is common, but physical signs are absent or minimal. The ESR is greatly elevated. Polymyalgia rheumatica is associated with temporal arteritis, and is sometimes the mode of onset of RA in the elderly. It is a difficult diagnosis, sometimes only confirmed by the dramatic, immediate response of both symptoms and the ESR to small doses of steroid (around 10–15 mg/day).

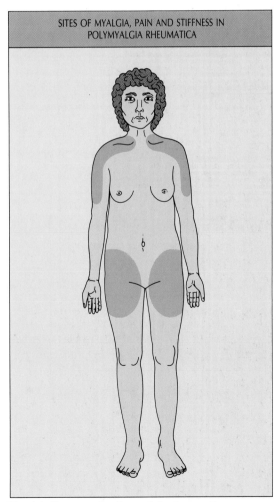

Fig. 13 *Joint involvement in systemic lupus erythematosus, and its common features.*

Fig. 14 *Pattern of polymyalgia rheumatica.*

Rheumatology is largely a clinical discipline. Investigations are of limited value, but may be necessary for one of three reasons:
- To confirm a diagnosis.
- To monitor the progress of a chronic disease, and/or the effects of treatment.
- To detect disease complications.

There are five main forms of investigation, each of which has a different role (Fig. 1). Other tests (imaging, arthroscopic examinations, tissue histology, etc.) are available to the specialist, but of little value in general practice.

Use, Abuse and Interpretation of Results

THE ACUTE PHASE RESPONSE: A variety of tests are available to screen people for inflammatory disease. Very high ESRs or the equivalent are common in active inflammatory polyarthritis and polymyalgia rheumatica. The CRP is often preferred by rheumatologists monitoring treatment of inflammatory arthropathies.

AUTOANTIBODIES: It is common to have low titres of a variety of autoantibodies, including rheumatoid factor. Only high titres are significant (greater than 1:128 for example, although this varies with different laboratories); a 'positive' test is of little value without the titre. Antibodies are often absent in early disease and false positives are common. Persistent high antibody titres correlate with more severe disease; however, it is wise not to rest a diagnosis on antibody tests, and much harm can be done by telling patients they are 'positive'.

SERUM URIC ACID: Some five per cent of the population have raised serum uric acid levels; very few of them get gout, and joint pains with hyperuricaemia is usually not gout. Hyperuricaemia on its own does not need treating. However, gout is rare in people with a normal/low uric acid level, and more likely if levels are high (above 0.5 mmol/l). Long term hypo-uricaemic therapy for gout should keep the levels below 0.4 mmol/l.

X-RAYS: X-Rays are one of the most useful tests in rheumatology. They provide an historical record of anatomical changes in joints that have occurred

INVESTIGATIONS IN RHEUMATOLOGY		
Type of Investigation	**Examples**	**Uses**
Assessment of the acute phase response	ESR Viscosity CRP	To see if there is inflammatory disease
Serum auto-antibodies	Rheumatoid factors Anti-nuclear factors	High titres suggest RA or SLE, respectively
Biochemistry	Uric acid	Gout
Imaging joints	X-rays	To detect the anatomical change in joints (often disease-specific)
Synovial fluid analysis	Polarized microscopy Microbiology	Crystal identification Septic arthritis
ESR = erythrocyte sedimentation rate CRP = C-reactive protein		RA = rheumatoid arthritis SLE = systemic lupus erythematosus

Fig. 1 *Investigations in rheumatology.*

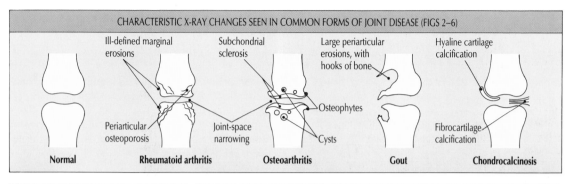

CHARACTERISTIC X-RAY CHANGES SEEN IN COMMON FORMS OF JOINT DISEASE (FIGS 2–6)

Ill-defined marginal erosions

Subchondrial sclerosis

Large periarticular erosions, with hooks of bone

Hyaline cartilage calcification

Periarticular osteoporosis

Joint-space narrowing

Osteophytes

Cysts

Fibrocartilage calcification

Normal   **Rheumatoid arthritis**   **Osteoarthritis**   **Gout**   **Chondrocalcinosis**

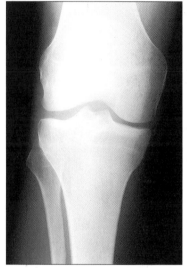

Fig. 2 *A normal, standing, anteroposterior X-ray of the knee joint.*

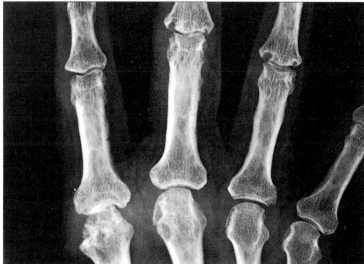

Fig. 3 *X-Ray of rheumatoid arthritis of the hand, showing erosions, joint-space narrowing and periarticular osteoporosis.*

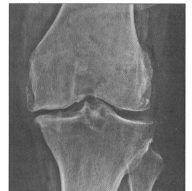

Fig. 4 *X-Ray of osteoarthritis of the knee, showing cysts, subcondrial sclerosis, osteophytes and joint-space narrowing.*

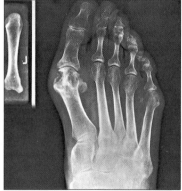

Fig. 5 *X-Ray of gout in the foot showing periarticular erosions with bone sclerosis and 'hooks'.*

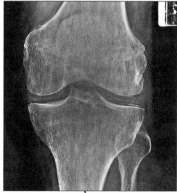

Fig. 6 *X-Ray of chondrocalcinosis of the knee showing linear fibrocartilage calcification.*

months or years previously. They are of little use in the acute stages of arthritis, but often show pathognomonic changes in chronic arthritis (Figs 2–6). X-Rays of the hands and feet are particularly useful in polyarthritis.

SYNOVIAL FLUID ANALYSIS: There are two circumstances in which synovial fluid is essential to confirm a diagnosis: crystal arthritis (gout and pseudo-gout) and septic arthritis. If an acute or chronic monoarthritis remains undiagnosed, synovial fluid should be obtained for specialist examination by polarized light microscopy (for crystals) and microbiology (Figs 7 & 8). The fluid should be sent to a laboratory as soon as possible, in plain sterile containers.

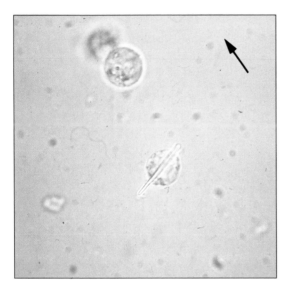

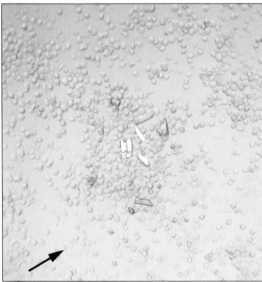

Fig. 7 *Crystals in synovial fluid viewed by polarized light microscopy: a typical negatively birefringent urate crystal attached to a cell (upper) and a cluster of positively birefringent calcium pyrophosphate dihydrate crystals in blood-stained synovial fluid (lower).*

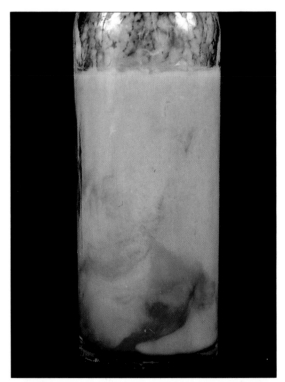

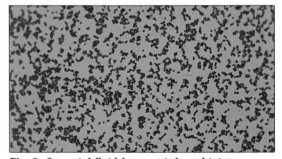

Fig. 8 *Synovial fluid from an infected joint (upper), which was shown to contain Gram-positive cocci (lower; courtesy of Dr D. Seal).*

Section 3

REGIONAL MUSCULOSKELETAL DISORDERS

THE HEAD AND NECK

Presentation

Disorders of the head and neck have acute or chronic presentations. Pain is the most common presenting symptom. Cervical root irritation causes pain, with a characteristic and often well-localized radiation. Diffuse pain arises from deep connective tissue structures, muscles, joints, bones and discs. Pain radiating to the back of the head is caused by upper cervical root irritation. Paraesthesiae and weakness in the upper limb suggest lower cervical root involvement. Neck pain is often accompanied by stiffness, and the consequent limitation of movement may extend to the shoulder, elbow and hand. Frozen shoulder, tennis elbow and carpal tunnel syndrome frequently accompany cervical spine syndromes.

Functional Anatomy

Neck pain may arise from articular and periarticular structures, or be referred (Fig. 1). The neck is the most mobile segment of the spine and is comprised of seven vertebrae united by intervertebral discs. This column is supported by a series of ligaments and the apophyseal joints between the spinous processes (Fig. 2). The articulation of C1 (the atlas) and C2 (the axis) is unique and prone to mechanical instability (Fig. 3). The intervertebral discs are made up of a tough outer ring (anulus fibrosus) and a soft central nucleus pulposus. Disc herniation is usually posterolateral and often results in pressure on the nerve roots at the exit foramina. The other periarticular structures giving rise to neck pain are the paraspinal ligaments. Many cervical abnormalities are perceived as neurological symptoms and signs in the upper limb, as C5 to T1 provide innervation to the entire arm. Pain may be referred to the neck from lesions of the shoulder, such as rotator cuff tendonitis, adhesive capsulitis and acromioclavicular arthritis.

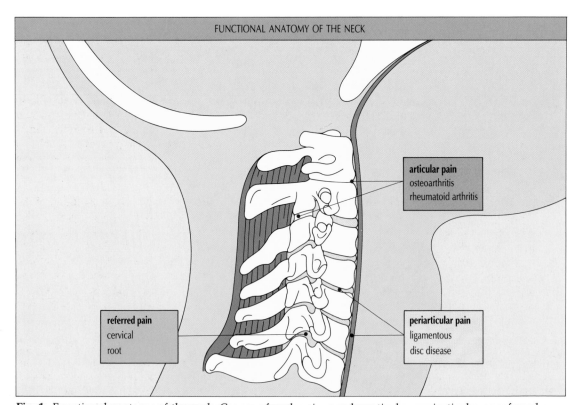

FUNCTIONAL ANATOMY OF THE NECK

articular pain
osteoarthritis
rheumatoid arthritis

referred pain
cervical
root

periarticular pain
ligamentous
disc disease

Fig. 1 *Functional anatomy of the neck. Causes of neck pain may be articular, periarticular or referred.*

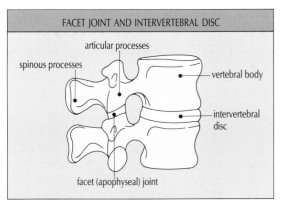

Fig. 2 *Diagrammatic representation of two vertebral bodies showing the facet joint and intervertebral disc.*

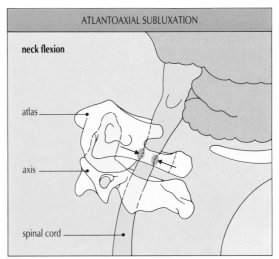

Fig. 3 *Atlantoaxial subluxation (schematic representation). If the atlas moves excessively on the axis, cord compression may ensue on neck flexion.*

Common Problems

- **Acute neck pain:** often follows a rotating or laterally flexing movement of the neck and results from injury and inflammation of the paracervical soft tissues.

- **Trauma:** most often a hyperextension–flexion (whiplash) injury following a road-traffic accident.

- **Chronic musculoligamentous neck pain:** damage and inflammation of the paraspinal ligaments and muscles.

- **Cervical spondylosis:** a combination of degenerative disc disease and facet joint osteoarthritis, this condition increases in frequency with age. It is a common cause of neck symptoms, but clinical features and radiological findings are often not related.

- **Spasmodic torticollis (wry neck):** usually a short-lived disorder in young people which resolves within a week.

- **Inflammatory arthritis:** rheumatoid arthritis, ankylosing spondylitis and juvenile chronic arthritis commonly involve the cervical spine.

- **Fibromyalgia:** see 'Pain All Over'.

Examination

It is easiest to examine the neck with the patient seated, and both upper limbs exposed. The examiner stands at the patient's side.

LOOK: at the position of the head and neck. These are not normally held stiffly to one side, or in flexion or extension. Swelling may be present in the supraclavicular fossae, anterior and posterior triangles of the neck. Look also at active neck movements and shoulder elevation.

FEEL: for tenderness of the bony structures of the neck. Posteriorly, these include the occiput, spinous processes of each vertebra, and facet joints. Although tenderness is a common finding in the absence of pathology, when localized over one vertebra it suggests bony pathology. Diffuse tenderness is more usual in musculoligamentous strains. Spasm of the sternomastoids and paracervical muscles is often palpable.

MOVE: to test flexion, extension, lateral flexion and rotation. Most cervical spine disorders are accompanied by some restriction of movement. Lateral flexion and rotation become affected earlier than flexion and extension. Discal pathology usually causes pain on flexion, while facet joint arthritis often causes pain on extension and rotation.

REFERRED PAIN: may occur in the arms, and neurological examination of the arms should be carried out. When arm pain is a result of nerve root irritation, symptoms may be reproduced by stretching the root (lateral flexion or rotation away from the side of the pain). The commonest roots to be involved are C2 and C5 (Figs 4 & 5).

Not to be Missed

- **Atlantoaxial subluxation:** resulting from inflammatory joint disorders, particularly rheumatoid arthritis, this can lead to laxity of the transverse ligament of the atlas with upper cervical cord compression by the dens of the axis (Fig. 6). Increasing neck pain and recent neurological deficit in the limbs of a patient with rheumatoid arthritis require radiological examination of the cervical spine in flexion and extension to rule out atlantoaxial subluxation. In addition, the complication may present with a variety of atypical neurological signs and symptoms.
- **Infection or malignancy:** can occur in disc spaces and vertebrae, which may become infected or be the site of bony metastases.
- **Osteophytic cord compression:** is an infrequent complication of cervical spondylosis in which exuberant osteophyte growth impinges on the spinal canal.

Investigations and Referral

Investigation and referral are unhelpful in the majority of cases. If an inflammatory cause is suspected, a full blood count, ESR and neck X-ray should be performed. Degenerative changes are common above the age of around 50 years, however, and may be irrelevant to the patient's symptoms. Requests for X-ray should thus be used sparingly in this group.

Patients should be referred if there is a suspicion of malignant disease or infection, or if neurological deficit becomes apparent.

Management
Acute Neck Pain

Acute episodes of neck pain can occur after injury or following specific movements such as extreme rotation. Pain is severe and accompanied by muscle spasm and loss of movement. Patients often require reassurance that the neck is not broken and relaxation therapy may be helpful. The neck is best supported in the position of least discomfort with a soft cervical collar. These may be obtained from a hospital appliance department or can be made by a practice nurse, using latex foam adhesive and tubular cotton. Analgesia and muscle relaxants are useful. Episodes usually settle within a few days but may be helped by physiotherapy, local heat and traction.

Chronic Neck Pain

This is the commonest type of neck pain in middle-aged and elderly people. Its natural history is variable, but pain is usually related to movement and the course is often punctuated by episodes of acute discomfort and muscle spasm. Pain results from a combination of chronic disc damage, facet joint osteoarthritis and muscle spasm. Neck physiotherapy, local heat, a soft cervical collar and analgesia form

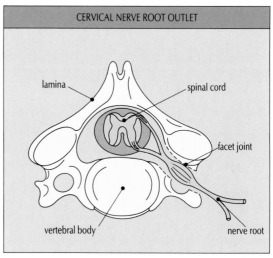

CERVICAL NERVE ROOT OUTLET

lamina — spinal cord — facet joint — nerve root — vertebral body

Fig. 4 *Anatomy of the cervical nerve root outlet. Note posterolateral exit foramen and proximity to facet joint. Facet joint osteophytosis often causes root irritation.*

the mainstays of therapy (although there is, in fact, scant evidence for the effectiveness of any of these measures). Reassurance, relaxation and advice on neck movements may also be useful. Intractable neck pain may be helped by acupuncture, transcutaneous nerve stimulation and anti-depressants.

CERVICAL ROOT LESIONS			
Dermatome distribution Anterior　　　　　Posterior	Root	Muscle weakness/ movement affected	Tendon reflex decreased
	C5	Shoulder abduction Elbow flexion	Biceps jerk
	C6	Wrist extension/pronation	Supinator jerk
	C7	Elbow/finger extension	Triceps jerk
	C8	Wrist/finger extension	Finger jerk
	T1	Finger abduction Thumb adduction/opposition	

Fig. 5 *Sensory and motor distribution of the cervical roots.*

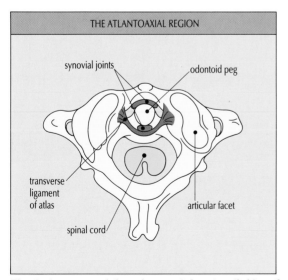 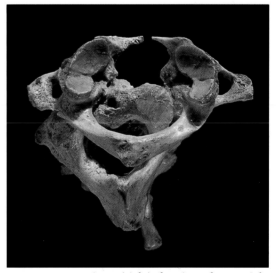

Fig. 6 *Anatomy of the atlantoaxial region (left) and a post-mortem specimen (right) showing atlantoaxial subluxation. Note the erosion of the odontoid peg, destruction of the anterior arch of the atlas, and posterior dislocation of the axis.*

LOW BACK PAIN

Presentation

Low back pain can be divided by onset and duration (acute and chronic), and by the quality and distribution of the pain (localized or with radiation) (Fig. 1). Acute, short-lasting episodes of localized pain are common, and may follow abnormal exertion or injury. The pain often radiates into the buttocks or top of the leg, but unilateral radiation below the knee and/or neurological symptoms suggests involvement of a nerve root. Chronic back pain of more than a few weeks' duration occasionally results from lack of resolution of the acute attack; more commonly it develops insidiously or with intermittent attacks of discomfort. Most chronic low back pain is classified as 'mechanical', being related to posture and movement, and localized around the back, buttocks and top of the legs. The pain may be referred from abdominal viscera or other structures, and is sometimes referred to the legs via nerve-root or cord compression. Severe morning stiffness with marked relief of pain by exercise suggests an inflammatory cause. New or 'different' pain in children and the elderly, and back pain accompanied by any systemic illness, may have a sinister cause.

TYPICAL LOW BACK PAIN DISTRIBUTIONS

● Tender spots: common in non-specific back pain, especially over paraspinal muscles (A) and on the pelvic brim (B)

● 1 Diffuse low back ache Common patterns in non-specific
 2 Diffuse buttock pain low back pain

 3 Diffuse pain radiating Common feature of apophyseal joint
 down the leg disease, sacroiilitis and non-specific
 back pain

● Localized central pain: uncommon, may indicate a sinister cause, especially if accompanied by severe localized tenderness

● Sharp pain radiating in well-defined area in the leg, often accompanied by paraesthesiae, indicates nerve root irritation

Fig. 1 *Some patterns of distribution of low back pain.*

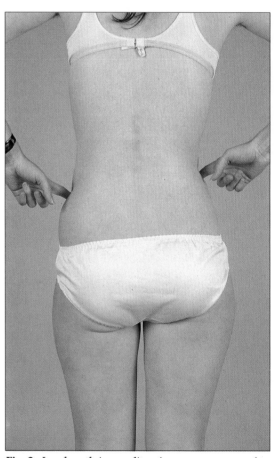

Fig. 2 *Leg length inequality. A common cause of non-specific mechanical low back pain.*

Common Problems

A precise diagnosis cannot be made in the majority of cases. Prolapsed intervertebral disc disease tends to be overdiagnosed, ankylosing spondylitis and sinister causes of back pain are often missed.

- **Mechanical low back pain:** episodic or chronic pain related to movement, made worse by prolonged sitting or standing, and often radiating into the buttocks and top of the legs. An extremely common symptom which may be exaggerated by anxiety, muscle tension or depression. A few cases have a clear mechanical cause such as instability, a spondylolysthesis or leg length inequality (Fig. 2). In some instances, local tenderness over ligament insertions suggests 'strain' to that ligament (for example, the ileolumbar ligament; Fig. 3).

- **Acute injury:** most common in young adults and those doing heavy work. Acute localized pain and muscle spasm usually resolve after a few days.

- **Spondylosis:** degeneration of the intervertebral discs and osteoarthritis of the apophyseal joints are universal over the age of 40. They sometimes give rise to symptoms, although there is no relationship between X-ray changes and pain severity. Disc disease causes back pain which is worst on bending forward or lifting. Apophyseal joint disease causes pain which is exacerbated by extension and often radiates into one or both legs, sometimes mimicking a 'slipped disc'.

- **Prolapsed intervertebral discs:** a distinct syndrome commonest in young adults and middle age. Usually acute low back pain is followed by radiation of severe pain with sensory symptoms in a nerve root distribution. Sometimes pain in the legs occurs on its own, without back symptoms. Coughing, sneezing and back movements can all cause 'shooting' pains in the legs. Neurological signs may develop.

- **Ankylosing spondylitis and related disorders:** these conditions are commonest in young men. They cause low back pain radiating into the buttocks and legs, worst in the mornings and often relieved by exercise.

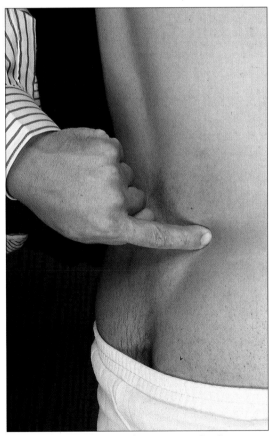

Fig. 3 *Palpating for tenderness over the ileo-lumbar ligament (a common site, sometimes responding well to local treatment).*

Functional Anatomy

The back is an extremely complex structure (Fig. 4). The anatomical origin of most back pain cannot be established, but mostly it is thought to arise from the ligaments and other periarticular supporting structures, and from the secondary muscle spasm that accompanies most back pain and 'splints' the spine. The disc spaces, apophyseal joints and sacro-iliac joints can all give rise to 'joint' pain, and disease of the vertebrae can cause 'bone' pain (Fig. 5). Pressure on the spinal cord or nerve roots from bony encroachment or soft tissues causes 'neurogenic' pain (Fig. 6).

Examination

It is easiest to examine the back with the patient standing and stripped to his/her underpants. Look and observe movement from behind the patient and then feel the spine and look for other signs with the patient on the couch.

LOOK: for any deformity of the spine including a scoliosis, exaggerated lordosis (often seen in mechanical back pain) or loss of lumbar lordosis (think of ankylosing spondylitis; Fig. 7). Look specifically for a pelvic tilt due to leg length inequality. A disc prolapse often results in an acquired scoliosis with visible muscle spasm.

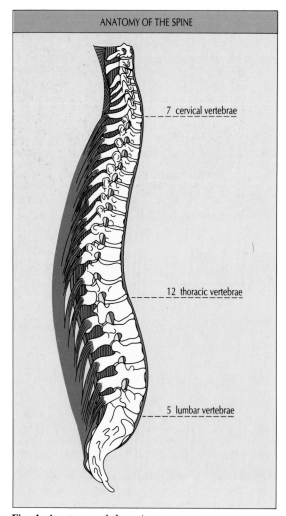

Fig. 4 *Anatomy of the spine.*

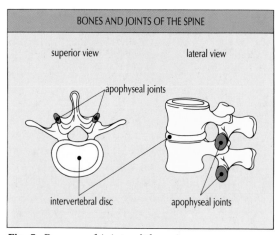

Fig. 5 *Bones and joints of the spine.*

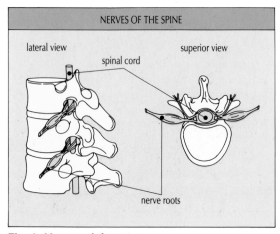

Fig. 6 *Nerves of the spine.*

FEEL: for any localized tenderness. Severe tenderness over one vertebra only suggests a sinister cause, but areas of tenderness around muscles and the pelvic brim are common whatever the cause of pain. Muscle spasm is often palpable and a spondylolysthesis is sometimes accompanied by a palpable 'step' between adjacent vertebrae (Fig. 8).

MOVE: Most organic back pain is accompanied by some restriction of flexion or extension. Ask the patient to touch their toes and arch their back fully. The degree of true spinal movement (as opposed to hip movement) can be observed and palpated by placing fingers over adjacent spinal processes (Fig.

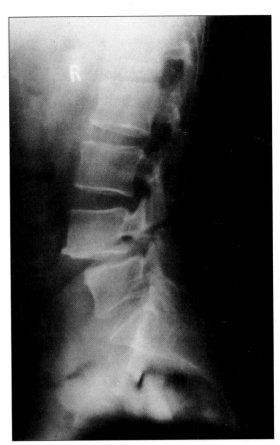

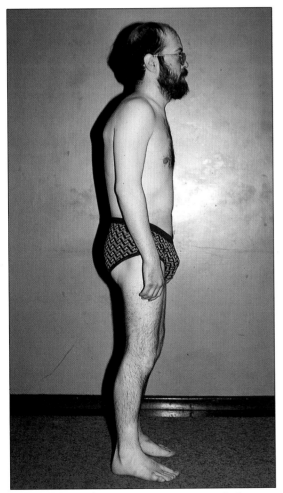

Fig. 7 *Loss of lumbar lordosis in early ankylosing spondylitis.*

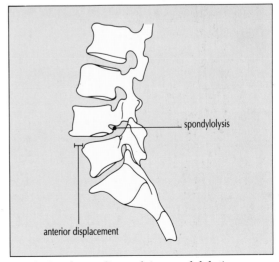

Fig. 8 *Lumbar radiograph in spondylolytic spondylolisthesis: a defect in the posterior elements at L4/5 has allowed the L4 vertebra to slip forwards on the L5 segment.*

3.9

9). Patients with specific mechanical abnormalities such as instability often 'climb up their legs' with the help of their hands as they straighten up. Look for loss of lateral flexion as well (symmetrical in ankylosing spondylitis, asymmetrical in a prolapsed disc).

REFERRED PAIN: The legs should be examined if there is any suspicion of disc prolapse or neurological problems. Sciatic and femoral stretch tests should be performed (Fig. 10), and the sensation and reflexes in the legs checked. The 'straight leg raising test' (SLR) is particularly important, helping to distinguish mechanical problems (back pain on SLR) from root irritation (paraesthesiae in the legs on SLR). An abdominal examination may be necessary to exclude referred pain from the stomach, pancreas, kidneys or other organs.

Investigations and Referral

Investigations are unnecessary and unhelpful in the majority of cases. Back pain should only be investigated in certain circumstances, and for exclusion of specific disorders.

If there is any suspicion of a sinister cause a full blood count, ESR and spinal X-rays should be performed. If ankylosing spondylitis is possible, a pelvic X-ray (to visualise the sacroiliac joints) and ESR should be done. If the back pain is unusually severe

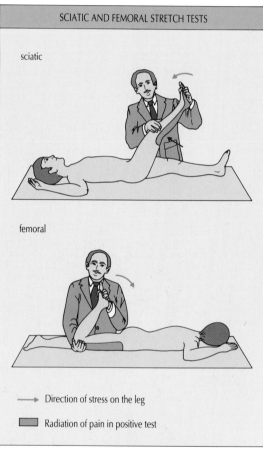

Fig. 10 Sciatic and femoral stretch tests. The patient should be resting, relaxed on a flat couch. The examiner gently lifts the leg as shown. A positive test results in sharp pain in the distribution of a nerve root due to pulling on the root which is under pressure. Some pain in the back, or in muscles such as the hamstrings, is common and must not be confused with a true positive.

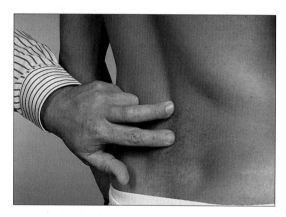

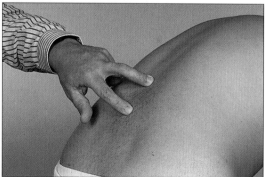

Fig. 9 Palpating for spinal movement. The examiner's index and middle fingers are placed over the palpable spinal processes of adjacent vertebrae. As the patient bends forward, the fingers move apart if there is movement between vertebrae.

or persistent, X-rays should be performed. However, interpretation of results is difficult. Early malignancy, infection, ankylosing spondylitis and other specific causes may not show up on the X-ray, and blood tests can also be normal. 'Degenerative' changes are very common and usually irrelevant.

Patients should be referred if there is a high degree of suspicion of a sinister or inflammatory cause; if there are any progressive neurological signs, any weakness, or any sphincter disturbance; and if the screening investigations are abnormal.

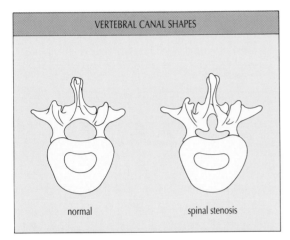

VERTEBRAL CANAL SHAPES

normal   spinal stenosis

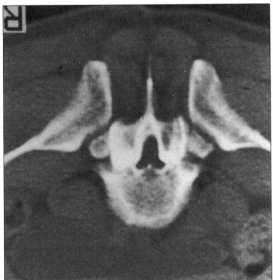

Fig. 11 *Spinal stenosis. The neural canal is narrowed due to congenital or acquired abnormality (eg. disc diseases); it is widest when the back is flexed.*

Not to be Missed

Most back pain is benign, mechanical and self-limiting. However, back pain is an occasional presentation of a large number of sinister disorders, and back disease occasionally results in significant neurological problems. Any progressive neurological problem or sphincter disturbance should be treated as an emergency.

- **Spinal stenosis.** Chronic disc problems and spondylosis sometimes lead to sufficient narrowing of the spinal canal to cause pressure on the cauda equina. The patient often presents with 'pseudo-claudication', leg pain brought on by exercise and relieved by rest, by sitting, or by bending forward (which opens the canal a little; Fig. 11). A variety of neurological signs may be present in the legs, and sphincter problems occasionally occur. Neurological signs may only appear after exercise.

- **Osteopaenia.** Osteoporosis (and occasionally osteomalacia) can cause vertebral fractures and can present as acute, episodic back pain, or with chronic symptoms. The thoracic, rather than lumbar spine is often maximally involved.

- **Infection or malignancy.** Disc spaces and vertebrae occasionally become infected, particularly in diabetics and others with reduced resistance to infection. Spinal bone secondaries may be the presentation of a tumour of the breast, prostate or other organs, and myeloma may present with back pain. Suspicious features include new pain in an older person, severe local bone tenderness, persistent night pain, and malaise, weight loss or fevers. Tumours in or around the spinal cord are an occasional cause of back pain with nerve involvement.

Management

The Acute Episode

Acute episodes of low back pain often occur after unaccustomed exercise, in association with a specific movement such as lifting, or after an injury. There is often severe pain, muscle spasm and loss of movement. The acute management is reassurance (patients sometimes fear they have 'broken their back'), alleviation of anxiety and muscle tension, rest in a position of least discomfort (often flat on the back on a firm mattress with pillows under the knees to flatten out the lumbar lordosis, or on the side with knees bent up), and analgesia, with or without muscle relaxants. Episodes usually settle in a few hours or days. Avoid prolonged bed rest. If the pain is persistent, consider physiotherapy with traction, manipulation and mobilization. Osteopaths and chiropractors often seem to be very successful in the management of acute back pain.

Chronic and Acute-on-Chronic Low Back Pain

Mechanical low back pain is an extremely common and difficult problem in middle-aged people. The division between acute episodes, chronic pain and acute-on-chronic pain is blurred. Look for a specific, treatable cause such as a leg length inequality or instability, even though nothing of this sort will be found in the majority of patients. Reassure that there is no serious problem, that it is not crippling, and that it is good to keep moving and active, even if there is pain. Consider whether depression, anxiety or some other psychological or social factor is contributing to the problem. There is no evidence that any specific treatment is particularly helpful, although patients should be taught back care and given advice about posture, chairs, beds, etc., to help them help themselves. Weight loss may be indicated. Patients complaining of severe pain need reassurance and relaxation, and they should be shown that they can move their backs by encouraging simple exercises (for example, gentle bending and rotation with encouragement to push just a little further each time).

Severe cases can be helped by back schools and back pain societies, by pain clinics, acupuncture, manipulators, transcutaneous nerve stimulation and antidepressants. It is important to encourage activity (aerobics, long walks with the dog, etc.) and independance, and to try to avoid medication, rest, corsets, referrals and time off work.

Prolapsed Intervertebral Disc

The typical history is of acute back pain (damage to the disc) followed either immediately or some hours or days later by referred, neurogenic pain in the distribution of one nerve root (due to the nucleus of the disc squeezing out onto a nerve root). Occasionally back pain is absent. Impulse pain and a positive stretch test are usual. Neurological signs may or may not be present; loss of sensation in a dermatome is the most common sign, loss of power or reflexes is less common and more worrying. The L4/5 space is most often involved, with signs in the L5 nerve root most common (Fig. 12). Treatment is initially as for any acute episode of back pain. Over 90% of cases resolve spontaneously within 6 weeks, but patients should be referred if they have persistent severe pain and/or progressive neurological changes.

Ankylosing Spondylitis

A disorder with a 4:1 male to female ratio. The onset is usually insidious and generally occurs in late teens or the twenties. Low back pain with morning stiffness, relief by exercise, and radiation of pain into the buttocks and back of the legs is usual. Many cases are erroneously diagnosed as slipped discs or non-specific back pain. Early signs include loss of the lumbar lordosis, limitation of lateral flexion, tenderness of the sacroiliac joints (a very non-specific sign) and some limitation of chest expansion (Fig. 13). Tender heels, red eyes or other features of the sero-negative spondarthropathies may be present, and a positive family history is common. X-ray changes only appear after the first few years of disease and the ESR is not always raised.

The pain and morning stiffness usually respond well to a night-time dose of a long acting non-steroidal anti-inflammatory agent, such as slow release indomethacin. This may help the diagnosis. However, the most important aspects of management are education and physical therapy. All patients should ideally be referred to a physiotherapy or rheumatology unit with knowledge and expertise, so that they can be taught how to keep their backs mobile and avoid late deformity (Fig. 14).

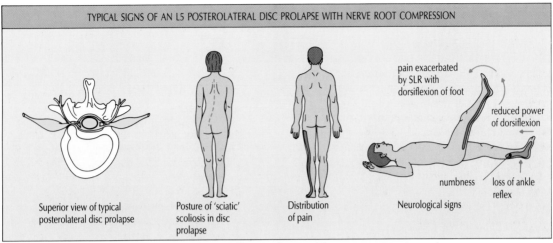

TYPICAL SIGNS OF AN L5 POSTEROLATERAL DISC PROLAPSE WITH NERVE ROOT COMPRESSION

Superior view of typical posterolateral disc prolapse

Posture of 'sciatic' scoliosis in disc prolapse

Distribution of pain

Neurological signs

pain exacerbated by SLR with dorsiflexion of foot

reduced power of dorsiflexion

numbness

loss of ankle reflex

Fig. 12 *Typical signs of an L5 posterolateral disc prolapse with nerve root compression.*

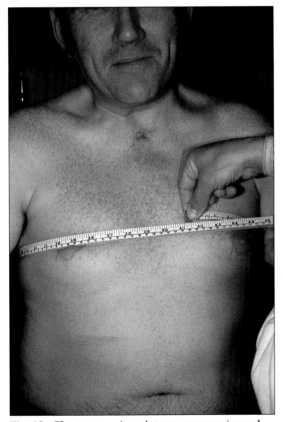

Fig. 13 *Chest expansion. A tape measure is used to measure the movement in full inspiration and expiration. A young man should have around 5cm of movement; less than 3cm is abnormal.*

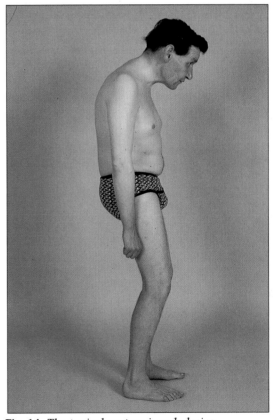

Fig. 14 *The typical posture in ankylosing spondylitis with the loss of lumbar lordosis, smooth thoracic kyphosis and a hyper-extended protruded neck. The hips and knees are slightly flexed.*

Presentation

Pain is the most frequent presentation of shoulder disorders. The nature of onset of the pain, and whether it was precipitated by acute or repeated trauma, helps to narrow down the cause. Common patterns of pain in the shoulder are shown in Fig. 1. Stiffness accompanies pain in intrinsic disorders of the shoulder, but is absent if pain is referred from pathology at other sites. Disability as a result of disorders of the shoulder is sometimes severe, and usually stems from inability to abduct and flex the joint.

Functional Anatomy

Pain in and around the shoulder may arise from the two main components of the joint (the glenohumeral and acromioclavicular joints), the periarticular structures (most notably the rotator cuff and sub-acromial bursa), and may be referred from the neck or heart (Fig. 2).

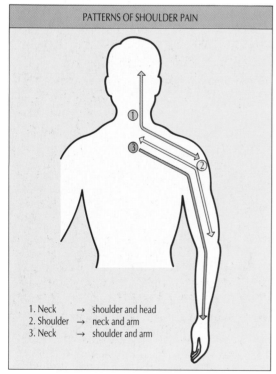

PATTERNS OF SHOULDER PAIN

1. Neck   → shoulder and head
2. Shoulder → neck and arm
3. Neck   → shoulder and arm

Fig. 1 *Common patterns of pain in the shoulder.*

Common Problems

- **Rotator cuff tendonitis and tears:** the rotator cuff (Fig. 3) is made up of four muscles (supraspinatus, infraspinatus, teres minor and subscapularis) whose tendons are incorporated into the capsule of the glenohumeral joint. These may become inflamed by repetitive use, or even torn by severe trauma.

- **Bicipital tendonitis:** inflammation of the biceps tendon as it runs along the bicipital groove on the anterior aspect of the upper humerus.

- **Adhesive capsulitis:** inflammation, followed by fibrinous adhesion, of the glenohumeral joint capsule resulting in a 'frozen' shoulder.

- **Subacromial bursitis:** inflammation of the subacromial bursa, which lies between the head of the acromion and the supraspinatus tendon, may result from over-use or an inflammatory arthritis.

- **Glenohumeral arthritis:** the shoulder is commonly affected by rheumatoid arthritis. Psoriatic arthritis and ankylosing spondylitis may also involve the shoulder. Septic arthritis must always be considered if only one shoulder is involved. Osteoarthritis very rarely affects the shoulders.

- **Acromioclavicular instability and arthritis:** inflammation of the acromioclavicular joint may follow trauma, such as a fall on the outstretched arm, and accompany inflammatory arthritis.

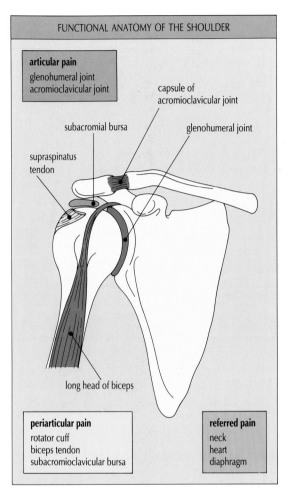

FUNCTIONAL ANATOMY OF THE SHOULDER

articular pain
glenohumeral joint
acromioclavicular joint

capsule of
acromioclavicular joint

subacromial bursa

glenohumeral joint

supraspinatus
tendon

long head of biceps

periarticular pain
rotator cuff
biceps tendon
subacromioclavicular bursa

referred pain
neck
heart
diaphragm

Fig. 2 *The functional anatomy of the shoulder.*

Examination

Examination of the shoulder is best carried out in two stages. Initially the region is inspected and palpated with the patient sitting facing the examiner. Ranges of active and passive movement are best assessed with the examiner behind the patient, so that scapular movement can be measured. A quick assessment of shoulder function may be made by assessing the patient's ability to raise their hands behind their head, and to hold their hands behind their back.

LOOK: for assymetry of the shoulders, indicating unilateral pathology. It may stem from deltoid muscle wasting or glenohumeral subluxation. Swelling is an

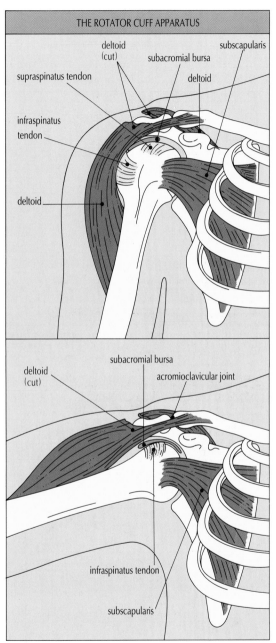

THE ROTATOR CUFF APPARATUS

deltoid
(cut)

subacromial bursa

subscapularis

supraspinatus tendon

deltoid

infraspinatus
tendon

deltoid

deltoid
(cut)

subacromial bursa

acromioclavicular joint

infraspinatus tendon

subscapularis

Fig. 3 *The rotator cuff apparatus. The tendons of the supraspinatus, infraspinatus and subscapularis pass between the top of the head of the humerus and the acromioclavicular joint. The subacromial bursa is also found in this region (upper).*
Abduction of the arm causes compression of the tendons and bursae and increases pain when the structures are inflamed (lower).

3.15

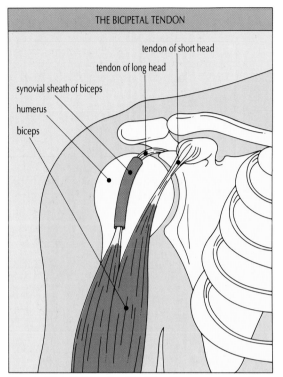
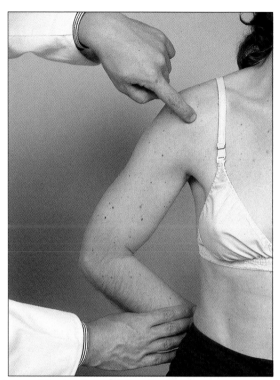

THE BICIPETAL TENDON

tendon of short head

tendon of long head

synovial sheath of biceps

humerus

biceps

Fig. 4 *Bicipital tendonitis. The diagram shows the anatomy of the tendon and the site that becomes inflamed over the head of the humerus. The examiner is palpating the tendon in its groove for evidence of local tenderness.*

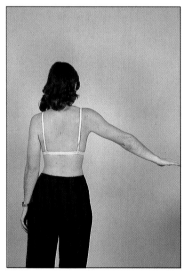
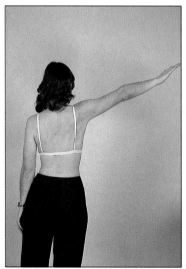
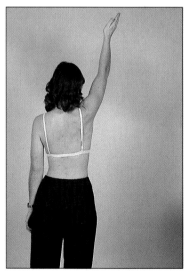

Fig. 5 *Inflammation of the subacromial bursa or rotator cuff tendons may cause a 'painful arc' during abduction of the shoulder). The initial movement (from the deltoid) is painless (left), but the next 90° of movement causes pain (middle). When the arm reaches full abduction (right) the pain ceases.*

3.16

unusual manifestation of glenohumeral disorders, but provides an important clue to acromioclavicular arthritis.

FEEL: for localized areas of tenderness. These are usually present in disorders of the subacromial bursa and biceps tendon (Fig. 4), as well as in acromioclavicular arthritis. Multiple tender spots around the shoulder are felt in fibromyalgia syndrome. In glenohumeral arthritis, tenderness around the joint is more diffuse. One or two tender spots around the shoulder, especially if symmetrical, may be normal.

MOVE: the shoulder actively and passively through its range of abduction–adduction, flexion–extension, and internal–external rotation. Abduction at the shoulder is divided into that which occurs at the glenohumeral joint (first 120°) and that which occurs at the scapulothoracic joint (subsequent 60°). Initiation of abduction depends upon supraspinatus contraction, with further elevation dependent on the deltoid.

Glenohumeral arthritis and adhesive capsulitis cause loss of active and passive ranges of movement in all directions, but most markedly in external rotation. Rotator cuff pathology sometimes causes a painful arc (Fig. 5), which progresses to limitation of active movement, especially abduction, but with preservation of passive movement. Acromioclavicular arthritis leads to pain at the extreme range of all passive movements. The acromioclavicular joint is stressed by pressing the patient's hand on the affected side against the contralateral shoulder.

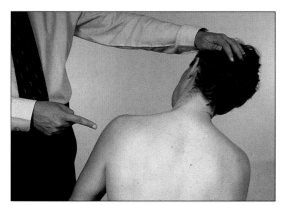

Fig. 6 *Referred pain from the neck is reproduced by moving the neck away from the side of the pain.*

REFERRED PAIN: in the shoulder arises most often from the neck and heart. If from the neck, pain follows the distribution of a cervical sensory root and is reproduced by moving the neck away from the side of the pain (Fig. 6). Motor abnormalities may accompany these sensory features.

Not to be Missed

- **The acutely painful, swollen shoulder:** arises from trauma, infection or crystal-induced arthritis. Traumatic damage may be limited to strain of the rotator cuff muscles or extend to fracture of the neck of the humerus. Infection of the glenohumeral joint is an uncommon but serious condition, often due to atypical organisms such as *Mycobacterium tuberculosis*. Chondrocalcinosis and concomitant pyrophosphate arthritis may also result in a painful, swollen shoulder.
- **Destructive arthritis of the shoulder:** progression of a monoarthritis of the shoulder to destroy the humeral head occurs in inflammatory arthritides, and also in association with deposition of calcium hydroxyapatite crystals (idiopathic destructive arthritis of the shoulder).
- **Bone lesions:** the most frequent to cause shoulder pain are multiple myeloma, secondary malignant deposits from solid tumours, and osteomalacia.

Investigations and Referral

Blood tests are usually unhelpful. Acute phase reactants often do not correlate with shoulder inflammation. Radiographic examination of the shoulder may show arthritis, calcific tendinitis, bony lesions and fracture, joint destruction and chondrocalcinosis.

Rotator cuff tendonitis and adhesive capsulitis are the most frequent shoulder disorders seen in general practice. These can usually be managed without referral. Hospital referral is required in the minority of patients with evident radiographic pathology, or in those who do not respond to the initial therapy provided.

3.17

Management
Rotator Cuff Tendonitis

Rotator cuff tendonitis is the most frequent peri-articular condition of the shoulder, and refers to a continuum of inflammation, degeneration and attrition of the rotator cuff, often triggered by trauma, and exacerbated by impingement on the undersurface of the acromion (Fig. 7). In a subset of patients the initial degenerative process is followed by secondary calcification in the tendon (calcific tendonitis). Early impingement is often seen in this group.

The initial management comprises physiotherapy (a graduated exercise regime, ultrasound and short-wave diathermy) and a local steroid injection (Fig. 8). The combination of local anaesthetic with the corticosteroid confirms precise localization of the lesion. Symptoms of rotator cuff tendonitis often recur after an initial response to injection. Repeated injections are often performed but specialist referral is appropriate at this stage. In rare instances of severe functional impairment stemming from rotator cuff tears or degeneration, surgical reconstruction may be attempted.

Bicipital Tendonitis

Tendonitis of the long head of the biceps often follows heavy lifting or strenuous activity. It leads to tenderness in the bicipital groove and pain on flexion

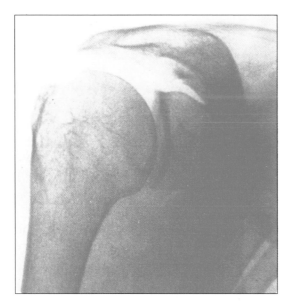

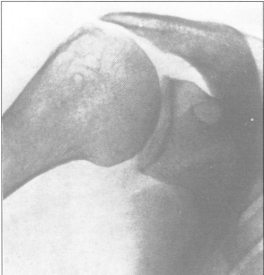

Fig. 7 *Xeroradiograph showing partial rupture of the rotator cuff. The head of the humerus subluxes upwards during abduction of the shoulder joint.*

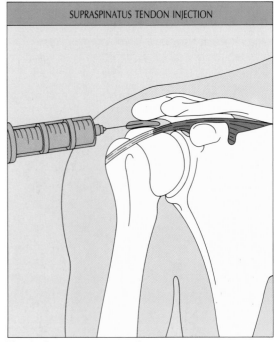

Fig. 8 *Supraspinatus tendon injection.*

and supination of the elbow. Rarely it progresses to rupture of the tendon. Physiotherapy with graduated exercises and ultrasound is the treatment of choice.

Adhesive Capsulitis (frozen shoulder)

The major articular disorder of the shoulder, this is a condition characterized clinically by pain and restricted passive movement at the glenohumeral joint. The pain is worse at night and external rotation is often markedly affected. It follows a classical time-course, with an initial phase of capsular inflammation lasting up to six months, during which pain is the major feature, followed by progressive capsular fibrosis, during which stiffness supervenes. The 'frozen' phase may last several months if untreated, but usually resolves spontaneously. Predisposing factors include previous rotator cuff tendonitis, diabetes mellitus and stroke.

The treatment of choice is physiotherapy. A local corticosteroid injection to the glenohumeral joint, via the anterior or posterior approaches (Fig. 9) may be helpful if the condition is encountered at an early stage.

Subacromial Bursitis

The usual cause is trauma or an underlying inflammatory arthritis and it presents typically as pain on active and passive abduction of the arm. It is treated by a corticosteroid injection into the subacromial bursa by a lateral approach.

Acromioclavicular Arthritis

An often unrecognized cause of shoulder pain, inflammation of the acromioclavicular joint accompanies inflammatory arthritides or follows trauma. It may be injected using a superolateral approach (Fig. 10).

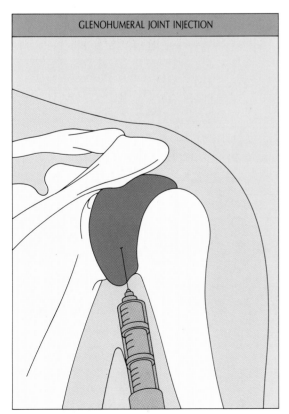

Fig. 9 *Glenohumeral joint injection.*

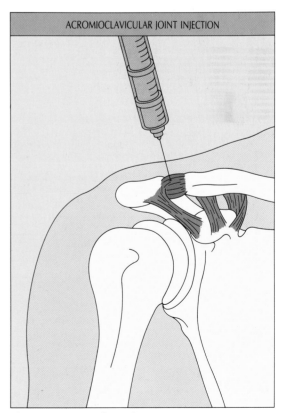

Fig. 10 *Acromioclavicular joint injection.*

Presentation

Damage to structures in or around the elbow usually presents as diffuse, poorly localized pain, radiating into the forearm (Fig. 1). It may be made worse by carrying or lifting and can be accompanied by sharp exacerbations of pain on movement. There may be a history of trauma or over-use. Patients sometimes present with 'lumps' on the elbow, with or without symptoms. Severe functional problems are an uncommon presentation or outcome of elbow disease, although pain on activity can prevent a sport or leisure pursuit (e.g. 'tennis' elbow). If elbow disease is accompanied by other problems in the upper limb — such as shoulder restriction — a significant handicap can result.

Functional Anatomy

The structures giving rise to pain in and around the elbow include the three main components of the joint (radio-ulnar, humero-ulnar and radio-humeral), the musculo-tendon insertions at the epicondyles and the olecranon bursa (Fig. 2). Pain can be referred from the neck and shoulder, or rarely from the heart or elsewhere (Fig. 3).

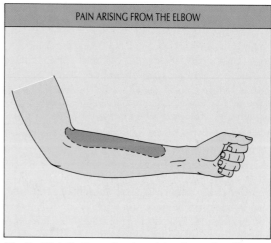

PAIN ARISING FROM THE ELBOW

Fig. 1 *Distribution of pain arising from the elbow. A diffuse ache which often radiates down the forearm.*

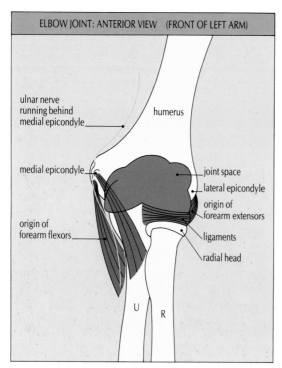

ELBOW JOINT: ANTERIOR VIEW   (FRONT OF LEFT ARM)

ulnar nerve running behind medial epicondyle

humerus

medial epicondyle

joint space

lateral epicondyle

origin of forearm extensors

origin of forearm flexors

ligaments

radial head

U   R

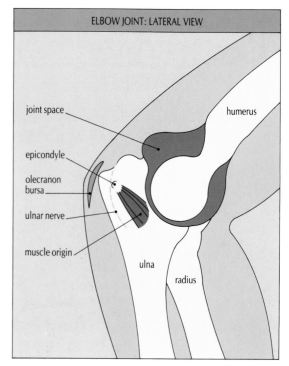

ELBOW JOINT: LATERAL VIEW

joint space

humerus

epicondyle

olecranon bursa

ulnar nerve

muscle origin

ulna

radius

Fig. 2 *Anatomy of the elbow joint.*

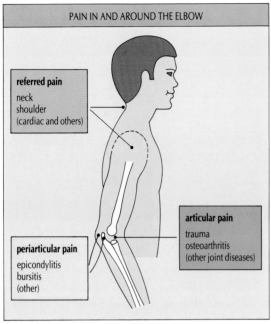

PAIN IN AND AROUND THE ELBOW

referred pain
neck
shoulder
(cardiac and others)

periarticular pain
epicondylitis
bursitis
(other)

articular pain
trauma
osteoarthritis
(other joint diseases)

Fig. 3 *Causes of pain in and around the elbow.*

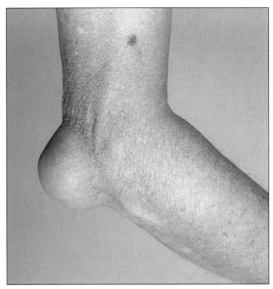

Fig. 4 *Olecranon bursitis. A soft, sometimes tender swelling over the tip of the elbow.*

Common Problems

Common causes of elbow/forearm pain include:

- **Epicondylitis:** damage and inflammation of the muscle origins at the lateral (tennis elbow) or medial (golfer's elbow) epicondyle.

- **Olecranon bursitis:** inflammatory swelling of the olecranon bursa on the tip of the elbow (Fig. 4). This can be due to over use (boozer's elbow), sepsis, crystals (e.g. gout) or an inflammatory arthritis.

- **Joint trauma:** damage to the bones, ligaments, capsule or intra-articular structures can occur with severe trauma.

- **Arthritis:** the elbow can be affected by osteoarthritis and many inflammatory arthropathies, although it is rare for them to present at the elbow, and there is usually obvious evidence of arthritis in other joints.

Examination

It is easiest to examine the patient seated, facing you, with both upper limbs fully exposed.

LOOK: for swellings around the elbow, especially over the olecranon, a common site for bursitis. Other swellings may be rheumatoid synovitis of the joint or rheumatoid nodules (they are hard lumps which are usually non-tender and generally lie under the skin, below the point of the elbow, and may be attached to the periosteum of the ulna; Fig. 5), in

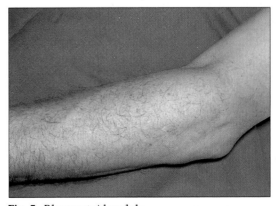

Fig. 5 *Rheumatoid nodule.*

which case the patient will generally have many other signs of rheumatoid arthritis. Gouty tophi, lipomas, xanthomas and others can occur, but they rarely cause symptoms.

FEEL: for localized areas of tenderness. In epicondylitis there will be highly localized, severe tenderness, which can be defined with one finger at or near the epicondyle (the precise point varies a lot) (Fig. 6). In arthritis there is usually more diffuse tenderness, which may be most marked over the radial head in line with the joint. Bursitis often causes local tenderness as well as the obvious swelling. If the pain is referred, no local abnormality can be found which will reproduce the symptoms.

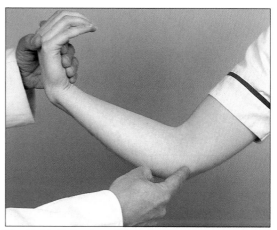

Fig. 7 *Medial epicondylitis (golfer's elbow). The tender spot around the medial epicondyle can be exacerbated by resisted flexion of the hand.*

elbow, and will be exacerbated by shoulder movement or stressing relevant tendons (e.g. the supraspinatus or biceps tendons — see 'The Shoulder').

Investigations and Referral

Tests add very little and referral is hardly ever necessary.

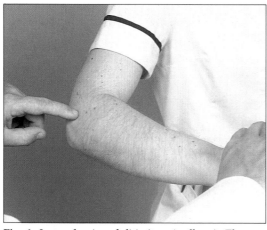

Fig. 6 *Lateral epicondylitis (tennis elbow). The tender spot can be defined with one finger. The pain is exacerbated by resisted extension of the hand.*

MOVE: the elbow through flexion and extension, pronation and supination. Arthritis usually causes loss of full extension (the patient may not have noticed this) and crepitus can often be felt. Epicondlylitis results in pain on resisted flexion or extension of the wrist (Fig. 7), which pulls on the damaged muscle origins.

REFERRED PAIN: may come from the neck or shoulder. If it is the neck (C5/6/7 roots) it is usually made worse when the head is moved away from the side of the lesion, and the neck itself may be stiff and painful. Pain from the shoulder can radiate to the

Not to be Missed

- **Olecranon bursitis** may be caused by infection or gout. If this is suspected fluid must be aspirated and sent for both bacteriological and crystal analysis. If sepsis has been excluded bursitis can be treated by injecting steroid and applying an elasticated tubular bandage.

- **Tenderness below the epicondyle** is sometimes present in normal people and can be severe in those with 'fibromyalgia' (see 'Pain All Over'). It is generally more diffuse, not clearly exacerbated by muscle use, and further away from the epicondyle than in a tennis or golfer's elbow.

Management

Tennis and Golfer's Elbow

These conditions arise from tears and inflammation at the common origins of the forearm extensors (lateral epicondyle — tennis elbow) or flexors (medial epicondylitis — golfer's elbow). They are common in young and middle-aged adults and are often due to injury or over-use. They may arise spontaneously, are rarely related directly to golf or tennis, and are never due to anything sinister. Pain on gripping, carrying and lifting can be severe and leisure pursuits are often affected. They can take months or years to resolve spontaneously. Recurrences are common — particularly if they are related to some specific activity.

MANAGEMENT: It may be best to try a splint first. A Laver splint is preferable; forearm splints can also be used (Fig. 8). This often prevents problems on activity by altering the pull on the muscle origin. Local injections are often necessary (Fig. 9). Drugs are of little use, although topical NSAIDs may relieve pain. Surgery is not always successful and should only be considered in the occasional very severe, unresponsive case.

Local injections should use about 0.5ml of a mixture of a depot steroid preparation and local anaesthetic. Identify the point of maximum tenderness, clean the area, and inject over it using a 'no-touch' technique and a 23 gauge needle (orange). The mixture should be infiltrated all round the maximum tender point, going down to bone. Local tenderness should be cured by the anaesthetic if the injection is in the right spot. Advise 48 hours rest of the arm after injection. Warn against the possibility of pain being worse in the first 24 hours and of local fat atrophy. Repeat once only if unsuccessful.

Note: you are safe around the lateral epicondyle, but the *ulnar nerve* runs just below the medial epicondyle. Be sure to keep well away from it by injecting from the other side (Fig. 7).

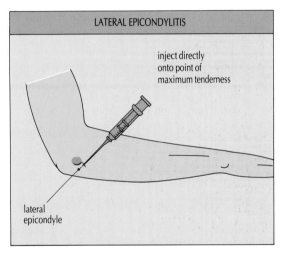

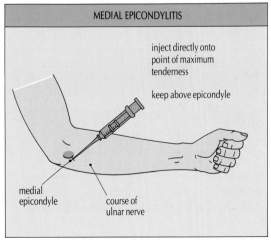

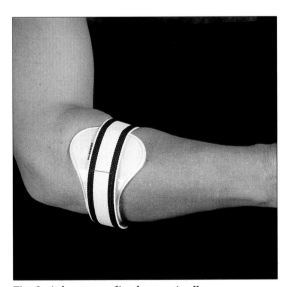

Fig. 8 *A forearm splint for tennis elbow.*

Fig. 9 *Injecting tennis and golfer's elbow.*

THE HAND AND WRIST

Presentation

The hands and wrists provide clues to the diagnosis of many rheumatic diseases. Disorders of the hand present in a variety of ways (Fig. 1). Pain may arise from several structures in the hand. Swelling and stiffness accompany pain in disorders of the joints and tendons. Paraesthesiae and paresis suggest local or distant neurological involvement. Raynaud's phenomenon is a frequent symptom in women and may indicate systemic connective tissue disease.

Loss of function is a critical feature in detection of hand disorders. It can result from mechanical obstructions as well as long-standing inflammatory joint disease.

Common Problems

Common non-traumatic problems occurring in the hands include:

- **Carpal tunnel syndrome:** entrapment of the median nerve as it passes beneath the flexor retinaculum at the wrist.

- **Flexor tenosynovitis (trigger finger):** inflammation of the flexor tendon sheaths. If the free passage of the tendon through the tendon slip is prevented, a trigger finger may result.

- **De Quervain's tenosynovitis:** inflammation of the tendon sheaths of the extensor pollicis brevis and abductor pollicis longus muscles.

- **Dupuytren's contracture:** a thickening of the palmar fascia that gives rise to usually painless flexion of one or more fingers.

- **Arthritis:** the hand is a common site for the presentation of a wide variety of arthritides. Most frequent among these are rheumatoid arthritis and osteoarthritis.

- **Raynaud's phenomenon:** a vascular disorder caused by episodic spasm of arterioles resulting in pain and triphasic colour change (white–blue–red) in the hands.

PRESENTATION OF DISORDERS OF THE HANDS	
Pain	Neurological symptoms
Swelling	Raynaud's phenomenon
Stiffness	Loss of function

Fig. 1 *Presentation of disorders of the hands.*

Functional Anatomy

Problems in the hand commonly arise from pathology in the joints, the periarticular tissues (especially tendons) and distant structures (leading to referred pain).

ARTICULAR: The joints of the hand are shown in Figure 2. Particular patterns of involvement of these joints are recognized in different rheumatic disorders. Rheumatoid arthritis tends to affect the metacarpophalangeal (MCP) and proximal interphalangeal (PIP) joints (Fig. 3). Osteoarthritis shows a predilection for the distal interphalangeal (DIP) and first carpometacarpal joints (Fig. 4).

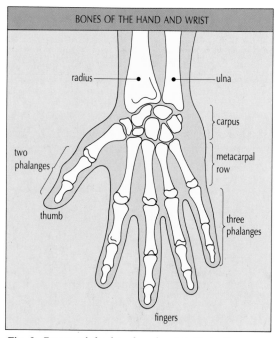

BONES OF THE HAND AND WRIST

radius — ulna

carpus

two phalanges

metacarpal row

thumb

three phalanges

fingers

Fig. 2 *Bones of the hand and wrist. Note the grouping of small joints: distal interphalangeal, proximal interphalangeal, metacarpophalangeal and carpometacarpal.*

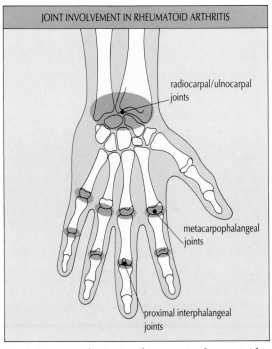

JOINT INVOLVEMENT IN RHEUMATOID ARTHRITIS

radiocarpal/ulnocarpal joints

metacarpophalangeal joints

proximal interphalangeal joints

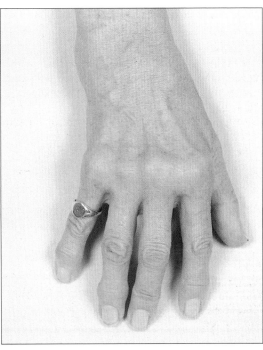

Fig. 3 *Pattern of joint involvement in rheumatoid arthritis. Note MCP swelling and radial deviation at the wrist.*

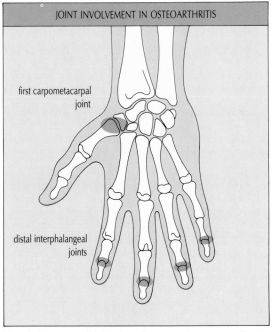

JOINT INVOLVEMENT IN OSTEOARTHRITIS

first carpometacarpal joint

distal interphalangeal joints

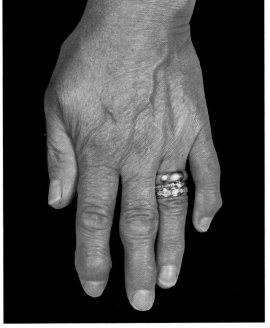

Fig. 4 *Pattern of joint involvement in osteoarthritis; note Heberden's nodes and squaring of first carpometacarpal joint.*

PERIARTICULAR: The flexors and extensors of the small hand joints insert into the phalanges through tendons. Inflammation of the flexor and extensor tendon sheaths (Figs 5 & 6) is a frequently encountered periarticular disorder. This may be generalized, as for example in inflammatory arthropathies, or well localized, for example to the extensor pollicis brevis following trauma or overuse.

REFERRED: Referred symptoms to the hand, predominantly pain, paraesthesiae and paresis, frequently arise from the cervical spine, compression of the ulnar nerve at the elbow, and compression of the median nerve in the carpal tunnel. The anatomical distribution of cervical roots in the arm is shown in 'The Head and Neck'; the sensory distributions of the median and ulnar nerves in the hand are shown in Figure 7. The motor supply to the small muscles of the hand is ulnar, except for abductor pollicis brevis, flexor pollicis longus, opponens pollicis and the lateral two lumbricals.

Examination

Examine the hands and wrists with the patient seated facing you. Most pathology can be discerned by exposing the hands and observing their palmar and dorsal surfaces at rest, and while closing and opening the fingers in a fist.

LOOK: for swelling around the joints, muscle wasting and deformity.

Swelling around joints may arise from synovitis (typically of the MCP and PIP joints in rheumatoid arthritis) or bone (Heberden's and Bouchard's nodes at the DIP and PIP joints in osteoarthritis). Swelling of tendon sheaths may be demarcated along their course, or be more diffuse. Oedema has many systemic causes but it does also occur in polyarticular inflammation. Other swellings occurring on the hand

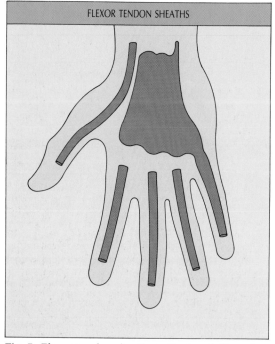

FLEXOR TENDON SHEATHS

Fig. 5 *Flexor tendon sheaths in the hand. Note the interrupted origin of the second, third and fourth digital tendon sheaths.*

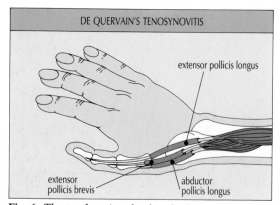

DE QUERVAIN'S TENOSYNOVITIS

extensor pollicis longus

extensor pollicis brevis

abductor pollicis longus

Fig. 6 *The tendons involved in de Quervain's tenosynovitis.*

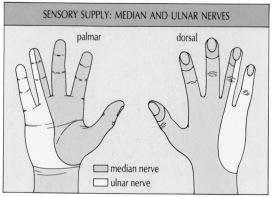

SENSORY SUPPLY: MEDIAN AND ULNAR NERVES

palmar   dorsal

☐ median nerve
☐ ulnar nerve

Fig. 7 *Sensory supply of median and ulnar nerves in the hand.*

include rheumatoid nodules (Fig. 8), ganglia, gouty tophi and xanthomata. Garrod's fatty pads (Fig. 9) often overlie the interphalangeal joints but do not signify any joint pathology.

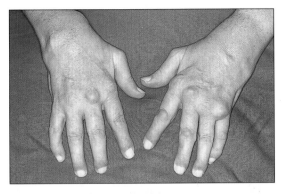

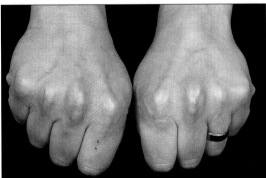

Fig. 8 *Rheumatoid nodules. These are present over the extensor aspect of the metacarpophalangeal joints.*

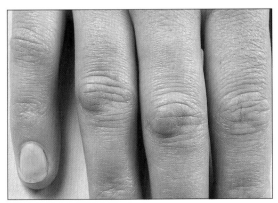

Fig. 9 *Garrod's fatty pads. Typical swellings over the proximal interphalangeal joints.*

Generalized wasting of the small muscles of the hand is a frequent sequel of immobility in rheumatic diseases; it may also occur in C8/T1 root lesions. Wasting confined to the thenar eminence suggests carpal tunnel syndrome (Fig. 10).

Deformity is a chronic sequel of joint disease. In long-standing rheumatoid arthritis, radial deviation occurs at the wrist with ulnar deviation at the MCP joints and subluxation at the MCP and PIP joints.

FEEL: for tenderness, for swelling, and for thickening of tendon sheaths.

Arthritis and tenosynovitis are usually associated with tenderness over the inflamed structure. Specific sites of tenderness should be sought which correspond with the joint patterns described above. Tenderness in the anatomical snuffbox can result from thumb-base osteoarthritis, inflammatory arthritis of the carpal bones and, if associated with trauma, from

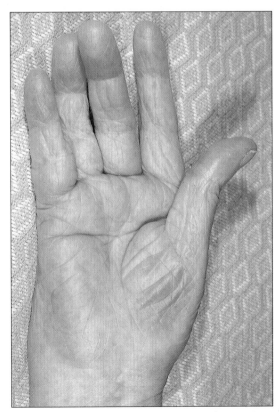

Fig. 10 *Carpal tunnel syndrome. Note the wasting of the abductor pollicis brevis and opponens pollicis.*

fractures of the scaphoid. The DIP joint osteophytosis which occurs in osteoarthritis is not tender.

Swelling arises from bone, fluid or soft tissue. Bony swelling is distinguished by palpation, though differentiation between fluid and soft tissue is more difficult.

Thickening of tendon sheaths is a common feature of subacute or chronic tenosynovitis and should be sought for in the extensor pollicis brevis and abductor pollicis longus tendons (De Quervain's tenosynovitis) and the long finger flexor tendons which are involved in triggering. Crepitus of the flexor tendon sheaths can sometimes be felt in tenosynovitis.

Neurological examination should not be omitted. In carpal tunnel syndrome, sensory deficit, found in the distribution of the median nerve, occurs with thenar wasting and weakness of abduction and opposition of the thumb (Fig. 10). Pressure over the carpal tunnel on the palmar aspect of the wrist, and

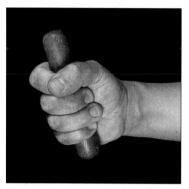
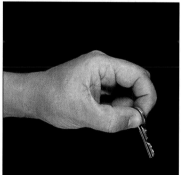
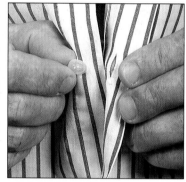

Fig. 11 *Assessment of function in the hand: grip (left), pinch (centre), fine movement (right).*

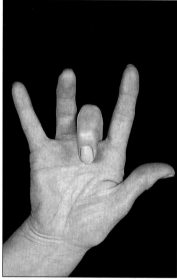
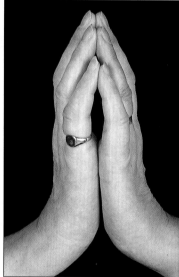
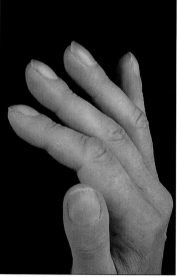

Fig. 12 *Trigger finger showing the ring finger caught in flexion. The patient was able to straighten the finger with force and an audible click could be felt.*

Fig. 13 *The prayer sign. The patient is attempting to place her hands in the prayer position but is unable to straighten her fingers.*

Fig. 14 *Hypertrophic osteoarthropathy. This patient with a bronchial carcinoma has finger clubbing and an oligoarthritis.*

active flexion of the wrist, may result in reproduction of neurological symptoms of median nerve irritation in carpal tunnel syndrome.

MOVE: the individual joints through their active and passive ranges of flexion, extension, abduction and adduction. Global assessment of hand function may be carried out by examining the ability to grip, pinch and perform fine movements (Fig. 11). Limitation of both active and passive ranges of movement is found in arthritis, while limitation of active movement with a normal passive range is more suggestive of a neurological disorder. Observe triggering of fingers during extension from the flexed position (Fig. 12). A sensitive indicator of arthritis or tenosynovitis is the 'prayer sign' (Fig. 13). Resisted movement in the direction of action of particular muscles is a feature of tenosynovitis.

REFERRED PAIN: usually arises from the neck or elbow. If cervical in origin, the pain is often worsened by moving the head away from the side of the lesion. If from nerve irritation at the elbow, neurological symptoms are often reproduced by pressure over the ulnar nerve.

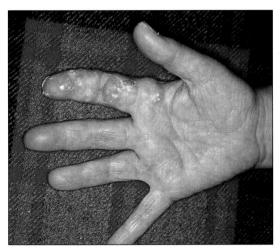

Fig. 15 *Calcinosis cutis: a large calcific mass in the index finger.*

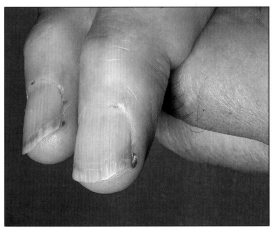

Fig. 16 *Rheumatoid vasculitis. Typical nail edge infarcts in a patient with rheumatoid arthritis, complicated by vasculitis. In the index finger there is also a small nailfold infarct.*

Not to be Missed

- **Transient postviral polyarthritis:** a variety of common viruses causing upper respiratory tract infections and skin rashes (adenovirus, herpes and enteroviruses) may cause a polyarthritis in young adults. This usually lasts a few weeks before resolving spontaneously. Long-term joint sequelae are infrequent.

- **Hypertrophic osteoarthropathy (HPOA):** clubbing of the fingers sometimes occurs as part of a syndrome in combination with proliferative periostitis of the long bones and an oligoarthritis (Fig. 14). Although uncommon, this syndrome may be associated with malignancy (particularly bronchial) and chronic infection. Pain and tenderness in HPOA are found near to, but not actually within, the joints of the wrist.

- **Scleroderma:** thickening of the skin of the fingers (sclerodactyly) occurs in connective tissue diseases, most commonly scleroderma. It may be associated with calcinosis (Fig. 15).

- **Vasculitis:** subungual splinter haemorrhages in patients with rheumatoid arthritis are suggestive of a systemic vasculitis (Fig. 16). This is a serious complication and warrants referral for specialist management.

Investigations and Referral

Haematological and immunological tests help to differentiate between inflammatory and non-inflammatory arthritis. Elevated ESR, plasma viscosity and C-reactive protein point towards an inflammatory disorder. Rheumatoid factor is present in 70% of patients with rheumatoid arthritis but also in 5% of the healthy population. Radiographs of the hands are useful in checking for erosions in inflammatory arthritis and for scaphoid fracture. Erosions are infrequent within the first 4 months of rheumatoid arthritis.

Management
Carpal Tunnel Syndrome

Compression of the median nerve as it passes beneath the flexor retinaculum often occurs in isolation but may be found in association with other conditions (Fig. 17). Characteristically, symptoms of median nerve irritation are worst at night and may be eased by shaking the hands. The condition usually commences unilaterally, but it progresses to the contralateral side in a substantial number of cases.

Initial management comprises use of a wrist splint (obtainable from an occupational therapy or physiotherapy department) and exclusion of associated pathologies. Drugs are of little use.

Second-stage management is a local steroid injection into the carpal tunnel (Fig. 18). This should be performed by an operator skilled in the procedure, as nerve injury is an infrequent but serious consequence of inexperience. Using a 23 gauge needle, the tunnel is entered from the palmar aspect

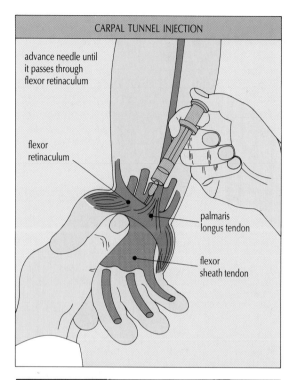

CARPAL TUNNEL INJECTION

advance needle until it passes through flexor retinaculum

flexor retinaculum

palmaris longus tendon

flexor sheath tendon

COMMON CAUSES OF CARPAL TUNNEL SYNDROME	
General	**Rheumatological**
Pregnancy	Rheumatoid arthritis
Diabetes mellitus	Other arthritides
Hypothyroidism	Tenosynovitis
Cardiac failure	

Fig. 17 *Common causes of carpal tunnel syndrome.*

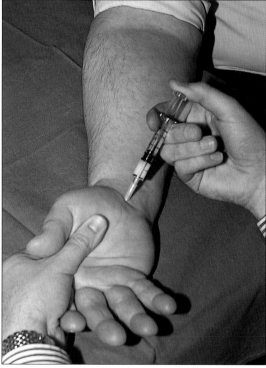

Fig. 18 *Injection of the carpal tunnel.*

of the wrist, just medial to the palmaris longus tendon, and level with the distal carpal crease; the needle is advanced until it passes through the flexor retinaculum (sometimes with a noticeable 'give'). Entry to the tunnel and subsequent injection of the steroid suspension often reproduces pain and paraesthesiae in a median nerve distribution. The wrist should be rested for 48 hours following the injection. Failure to resolve following injection, or the onset of muscle wasting, are indications to consider carpal tunnel release.

Trigger Finger

Trigger fingers result from a nodular or stenosing tenosynovitis of the finger flexors, giving rise to a mechanical obstruction on flexing or extending the affected finger. They are efficiently treated by local steroid injections, the results of which are good; but in the few cases which do not resolve, surgery may be necessary.

De Quervain's Tenosynovitis

Tenosynovitis of the extensor pollicis brevis and abductor pollicis longus may be helped by injection, with a mixture of corticosteroid and local anaesthetic (Fig. 19). The needle is inserted at a 45° angle over the palmar aspect of the affected metacarpal head and is advanced proximally almost parallel to the skin and the mixture infiltrated proximally. Failure to resolve after injection is an indication for surgical release.

Raynaud's Phenomenon

Classic Raynaud's phenomenon (Fig. 20) manifests as a three-phase change in hand colour, precipitated by exposure to cold. The initial pallor comes from arterial constriction, and is followed by cyanosis resulting from deoxygenation of haemoglobin in dermal capillaries, and then hyperaemia as the vessels dilate and refill with arterial blood. About 10% of patients with Raynaud's phenomenon have some other underlying abnormality; most frequent among these are connective tissue diseases (especially systemic sclerosis), thoracic outlet syndromes, arterial diseases and haematological disorders (such as cryoglobulinaemia).

Treatment involves excluding an underlying disorder and avoidance of the precipitating stimulus

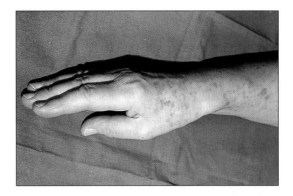

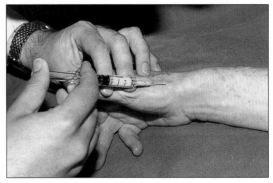

Fig. 19 *Injection of de Quervain's tenosynovitis.*

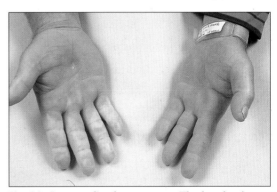

Fig. 20 *Raynaud's phenomenon. The hands of a patient with severe Raynaud's phenomenon showing the typical white appearance of the fingers. The left index finger has been amputated due to previous gangrene.*

(cold). Various drugs have been tried with limited success, including calcium channel blockers and vasodilators. Surgery to the sympathetic nervous system is possible but not required in most patients.

Presentation

Patients will often use the expression 'hip pain' to refer to pain anywhere from the iliac crest and buttock to the greater trochanter and thigh. As locating the exact site of pain is useful in determining the cause, it is important to ask the patient to point to the painful area (Fig. 1). Pain due to hip-joint disease is usually felt in the groin but is also sometimes felt in the buttock, over the greater trochanter, in the thigh or at the knee. Soft tissue lesions around the hip and lumbar spine disease also commonly present with pain in these regions, but in most cases the source of pain can be determined from a careful examination. A limp may be found in the presence of hip disease and can occur without pain.

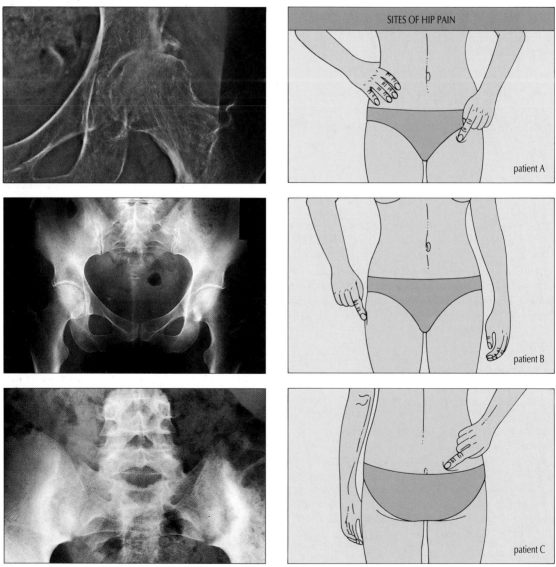

SITES OF HIP PAIN

patient A

patient B

patient C

Fig. 1 *All three of these patients presented with hip pain. When asked to indicate the maximal site of pain, patient A (osteoarthritis of the hip) indicated the groin, patient B (trochanteric bursitis; note normal X-ray) the greater trochanter, and patient C (sacroiliitis) the buttock.*

Common Problems

Common causes of pain around the hip include:

- **Arthritis:** osteoarthritis is the commonest type of hip disease (see 'Management', below). Inflammatory arthritides (such as rheumatoid arthritis) may involve the hip but usually only after extensive involvement of other joints. In ankylosing spondylitis, hip disease often occurs in the absence of other peripheral joint involvement. The combination of a stiff hip and spine produces a major functional problem (Fig. 2).
- **Lumbar spine disease:** this is a frequent and troublesome cause of 'hip' pain (see 'Referred Pain', below).
- **Trochanteric bursitis:** is a common cause of pain in the region of the greater trochanter (see 'Management', below). Ischial bursitis (a much less frequent problem) causes pain over the ischial tuberosity.
- **Polymyalgia rheumatica:** although shoulder girdle symptoms usually predominate, bilateral hip pain associated with prominent morning stiffness in a patient over 60 years old could be polymyalgia rheumatica (see 'Pain All Over').
- **Irritable hip (children):** hip pain and/or a limp in children warrants referral to a hospital specialist. Irritable hip, otherwise known as transient synovitis of the hip, is a syndrome of unknown cause, producing a limp and pain in the hip for a period of a few weeks. Paediatric referral may be helpful as the diagnosis must only be made after exclusion of more serious hip disorders: infection, congenital dislocation, Perthes' disease and slipped capital epiphysis (Fig. 3).
- **Tendon-related symptoms:** pain at the insertion of the adductor tendon onto the pelvis is most often due to over-use in athletes, but this area may also become inflamed in the seronegative spondyloarthropathies, such as ankylosing spondylitis.

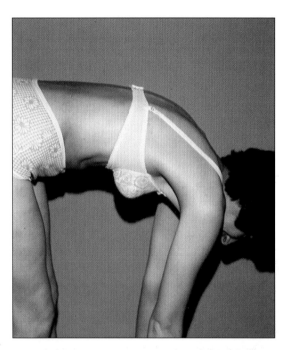

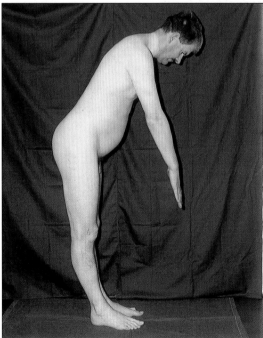

Fig. 2 *Both these patients with ankylosing spondylitis have rigid spines. The woman has normal hips and can still touch her toes; the man has stiff hips and consequently has major functional disability.*

3.33

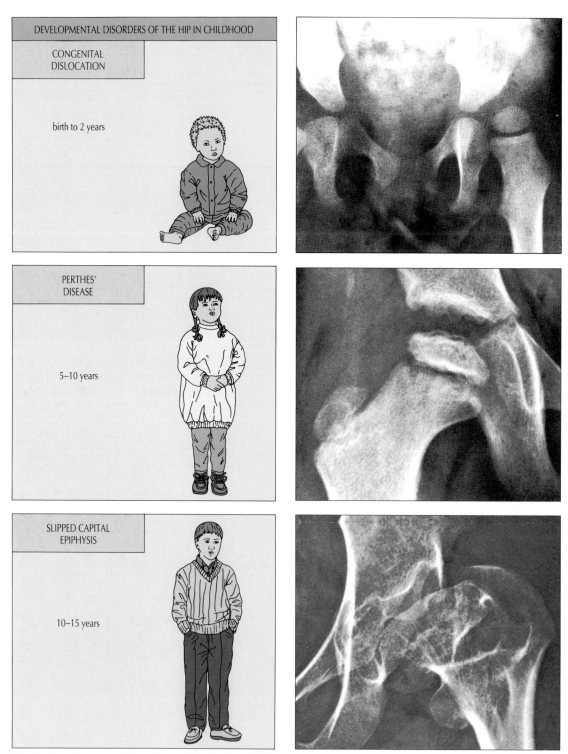

DEVELOPMENTAL DISORDERS OF THE HIP IN CHILDHOOD

CONGENITAL DISLOCATION

birth to 2 years

PERTHES' DISEASE

5–10 years

SLIPPED CAPITAL EPIPHYSIS

10–15 years

Fig. 3 *Developmental disorders of the hip in childhood.*

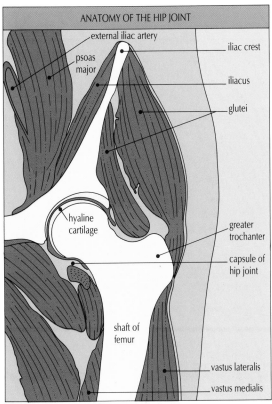

Fig. 4 *Anatomy of the hip joint.*

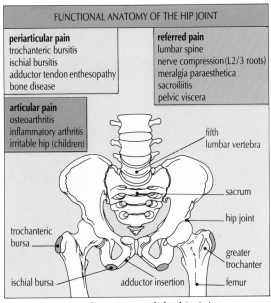

Fig. 5 *Functional anatomy of the hip joint.*

Functional Anatomy

Pain in the region of the hip may arise from the hip joint, bursae, tendon insertions, sacroiliac joints, bone of femur or pelvis, intrapelvic viscera, abdominal wall (for example, herniae) or the lumbar spine and its associated nerve roots (Figs 4 & 5).

Examination

The patient should be examined in underwear only, so that the iliac crests and the spine are visible. Watching the patient walk will provide useful information about overall function.

LOOK: at the patient from behind, with the patient standing, to see if there is any buttock wasting, pelvic tilt or lumbar scoliosis (as may occur secondary to hip disease). Watch the patient walking, noting any gait abnormality.

FEEL: for specific tender sites. This is the most important clinical sign for periarticular problems such as trochanteric and ischial bursitis, and adductor enthesitis. Tenderness arising from pathology in the hip joint tends to be anterior, and medial to the femoral pulse (Fig. 6).

MOVE: the hip as described below. Articular disease will result in restricted painful movement. Inflamed

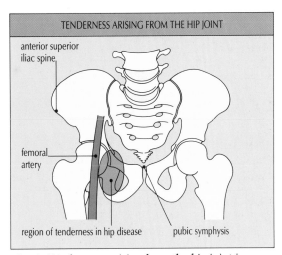

Fig. 6 *Tenderness arising from the hip joint is usually anterior, and medial to the femoral pulse.*

3.35

or damaged hips are often held in flexion. By fully flexing the contralateral hip any forward pelvic tilt can be abolished, and if the ipsilateral hip is unable to fully extend the thigh will be seen to lift off the couch (Thomas test, Fig. 7). Abduction and adduction are best assessed with the knee extended, rotation and flexion with the knee flexed (Fig. 8). Loss of internal rotation is a particularly important sign as it occurs early in diseases of the hip joint.

REFERRED PAIN: over the lateral and anterior aspects of the thigh (see 'Low Back Pain') is frequently caused by lumbar spine disease and sacroiliitis, usually in the form of degenerative spondylosis. Irritation or compression of the lateral cutaneous nerve of the thigh (meralgia paraesthetica), or the L2/3 nerve roots from which it derives, produces pain, hyperalgesia and paraesthesia over the lateral aspect of the thigh. In all these conditions, passive hip rotation is normal and pain-free, a sign which distinguishes them from hip disease.

Not to be Missed

- **Infection** involving the hip or sacroiliac joint is rare and difficult to recognize. Suspect it when pain is constant and progressive and the patient is unwell. (See 'The Acutely Painful Joint'.)
- **Bone diseases** such as tumours, ischaemic necrosis (Fig. 9), Paget's disease and fracture may present with pain that is usually diffuse and constant.
- **Intrapelvic visceral and arterial disease** may cause pain referred to the hip or buttock.

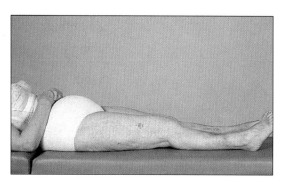

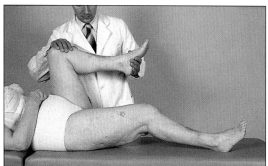

Fig. 7 *Thomas test. The patient has osteoarthritis of the right hip which lacks extension (a fixed flexion deformity). The patient is able to lie flat on the couch due to a compensatory lumbar lordosis (upper). When the normal, left hip is fully flexed by the examiner the lumbar lordosis is overcome by pelvic rotation and the fixed flexion deformity is unmasked, the right leg then lifting from the couch (lower).*

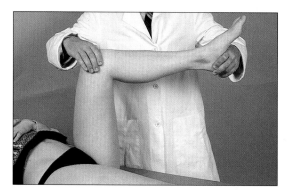

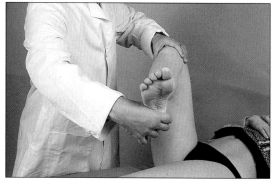

Fig. 8 *Assessing internal (upper) and external (lower) rotation of the hip. The leg acts as a pointer which shows the angle of rotation.*

Investigations and Referral

X-ray is the single most useful investigation. Significant chronic arthritis of the hip, Paget's disease and bone tumours will usually be detected. ESR will usually be elevated in polymyalgia rheumatica, and often in inflammatory arthritis. Although useful when raised, it should be noted that a normal blood white-cell count and ESR do not exclude septic arthritis of the hip. Aspiration and injection of the hip joint is difficult and is usually performed under X-ray guidance.

Management

Osteoarthritis

Although occasionally there is an identifiable cause, such as congenital dislocation or acetabular dysplasia, usually no cause is apparent for this common problem. Progression is difficult to predict. Although some patients may deteriorate rapidly, the disease often appears to remain stable for many years. Treatment in the majority consists of regular simple analgesia (such as paracetemol) and advice to 'keep moving'. Swimming and walking are good exercises. A walking stick held in the opposite hand will unload about a quarter of the weight on the hip and so should be encouraged. Weight reduction may also

relieve pain. Physiotherapy (with hydrotherapy), occupational therapy assessment (see Section 5) or a short course of a non-steroidal anti-inflammatory drug often helps. A minority of patients will require surgery (usually total hip replacement). New hip pain following a total hip replacement is an indication for urgent orthopaedic referral, as it may signify loosening of the prosthesis or infection.

Trochanteric Bursitis

Inflammation of any of the trochanteric bursae (which separate the tendons of gluteus medius, minimus and maximus from the trochanter) gives rise to pain which is frequently most troublesome at night and may prevent the patient lying on the affected side. Climbing stairs and walking may also be painful even though the range of passive motion of the hip is normal on examination. The key sign is tenderness present over or just posterior to the greater trochanter. When this sign is present, treatment of trochanteric bursitis is worthwhile even if the patient also has osteoarthritis. Treatment consists of local heat and, if necessary, an injection of local anaesthetic and a depot steroid preparation given at the site of maximum tenderness. The needle should be introduced deeply – if the periosteum is reached, withdraw a couple of millimetres then inject slowly. There should be little resistance to injection. A repeat injection after a few weeks is sometimes required.

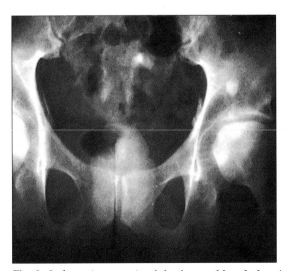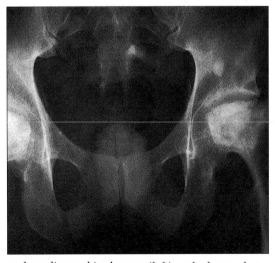

Fig. 9 *Ischaemic necrosis of the femoral head, showing early radiographic changes (left) and advanced changes (right). Courtesy of Professor M. Kahn.*

Presentation

The common presenting symptoms for patients with problems in and around the knee are pain in the knee, limping and a feeling of insecurity on walking ('the knee feels as if it might give way'). A history of trauma and meniscectomy many years earlier may point to osteoarthritis as the cause. Anterior knee pain (felt just deep to the patella), particularly in a young woman, suggests patellofemoral problems, but localized anterior pain may be due to a peri-articular problem (e.g. bursitis, Fig. 1). Diffuse knee pain usually results from arthritis of the knee or hip. Locking is a common symptom, but only a minority of these patients have true locking (intermittent inability to move the joint due to a mechanical block, not just an unwillingness to move due to pain) which, when it is present, suggests an intra-articular loose body or torn meniscus.

Functional Anatomy

Pain in the knee may arise from any of the three main compartments of the joint (medial and lateral tibiofemoral and patellofemoral), the bursae, menisci, ligaments or their insertions (Fig. 2). Pain may also be referred from the hip or lumbar spine (L3,4,5) (Fig. 3).

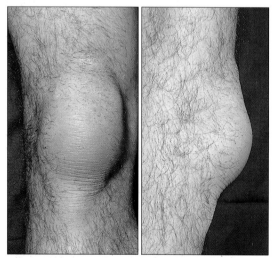

Fig. 1 *Prepatellar bursitis: anterior (left) and lateral (right) view of a red, swollen, painful prepatellar bursa.*

Common Problems

Common causes of knee pain include:
- **Arthritis:** osteoarthritis of the knee is very common especially in women and older people. Inflammatory arthritides, such as rheumatoid arthritis, frequently involve the knee and occasionally present with isolated involvement of one or both knees.
- **Trauma:** soft tissue injuries of the knee include torn menisci, cruciate and collateral ligamentous tears, and traumatic synovitis. Careful assessment of the severity of the trauma and its relationship to symptoms is required as patients frequently inappropriately relate joint problems to minor trauma.
- **Anterior knee pain** (e.g. chondromalacia patellae): usually worse on the stairs, and occurring most commonly in teenage girls, this is a symptom complex that is sometimes associated with fissuring of the cartilage on the undersurface of the patella (chondromalacia patellae) or with abnormal tracking of the patellofemoral apparatus, but often no definable abnormality is present.
- **Bursitis:** prepatella bursitis (housemaid's knee; Fig. 1) and infrapatella bursitis (clergyman's knee) usually relate to minor repetitive trauma and result in thickening of the wall of the involved bursa with effusion. If the skin overlying the bursa is red, hot and tender, a superimposed infection should be excluded although usually this lesion is non-infective.

Examination

Careful inspection of the patient's gait and erect stance will provide useful clues (Fig. 4). Formal examination is easiest if the patient (in underwear only) lies supine on a couch.

LOOK: for deformity of the knee, which is best seen with the patient standing. Although exceptions are common, osteoarthritis tends to produce varus, and rheumatoid arthritis valgus, deformities at the knee (Fig. 5). A surgical scar over the joint may indicate

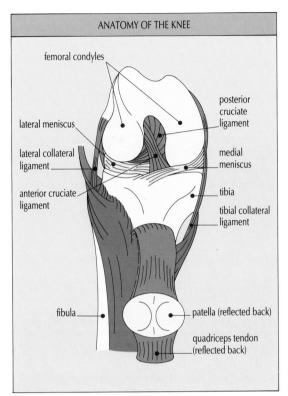

ANATOMY OF THE KNEE

femoral condyles
posterior cruciate ligament
lateral meniscus
medial meniscus
lateral collateral ligament
anterior cruciate ligament
tibia
tibial collateral ligament
fibula
patella (reflected back)
quadriceps tendon (reflected back)

Fig. 2 *Anatomy of the right knee joint from the front (with the knee bent).*

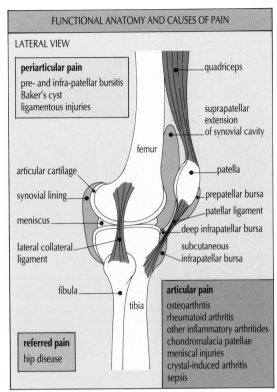

FUNCTIONAL ANATOMY AND CAUSES OF PAIN

LATERAL VIEW

periarticular pain
pre- and infra-patellar bursitis
Baker's cyst
ligamentous injuries

quadriceps
suprapatellar extension of synovial cavity
femur
articular cartilage
patella
synovial lining
prepatellar bursa
meniscus
patellar ligament
deep infrapatellar bursa
lateral collateral ligament
subcutaneous infrapatellar bursa
fibula
tibia

articular pain
osteoarthritis
rheumatoid arthritis
other inflammatory arthritides
chondromalacia patellae
meniscal injuries
crystal-induced arthritis
sepsis

referred pain
hip disease

Fig. 3 *Functional anatomy and causes of pain in and around the knee.*

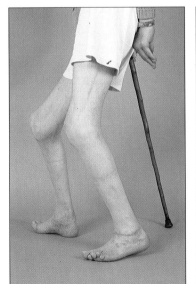

Fig. 4 *Examination of gait is an essential part of examination.*

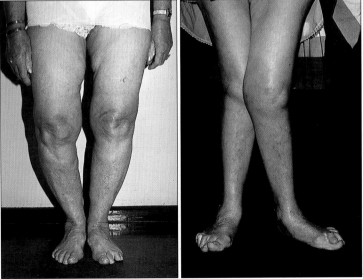

Fig. 5 *Osteoarthritis tends to produce varus (left) and rheumatoid arthritis valgus (right) deformity of the knee.*

previous trauma and/or meniscectomy. Infra- and prepatellar bursitis will produce prominent swelling anterior to the knee, often associated with erythema, usually in the absence of a true joint effusion. A Baker's cyst may be more easily seen than felt (Fig. 6).

FEEL: to determine whether swelling is soft (effusion or synovial thickening) or hard (bone or cartilage). Hard swelling suggests osteoarthritis, although inflammatory arthropathies may also produce hard swelling in the later stages due to secondary osteo-

arthritic changes. Quadriceps wasting occurs with all forms of knee disease and can be seen or felt (Fig. 7). Small effusions of the knee are best tested for by attempting to move fluid from one side of the joint to the other (the bulge sign; Fig. 8), whereas larger effusions are most easily detected by the presence of a patellar tap (Fig. 9). Tenderness is frequently present around the joint line in osteoarthritis, whereas generalized tenderness is more commonly found in inflammatory arthritis. Tenderness of the subcutaneous fat on the medial side of the knee is common, especially in obese women, and may occur in the absence of arthritis.

MOVE: to determine the range of motion, feel for crepitus and check for ligament instability (Figs 10 & 11). A small loss of extension (i.e. a fixed flexion deformity) will prevent the patient locking the knee during normal walking and represents a much more

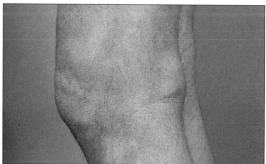

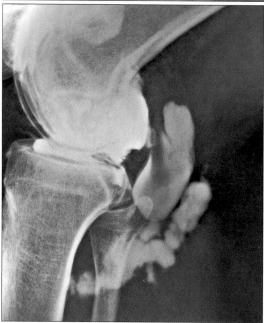

Fig. 6 *Clinical view of a Baker's cyst (upper), and an arthrogram demonstrating a ruptured cyst (lower) where the fluid has leaked into the soft tissues.*

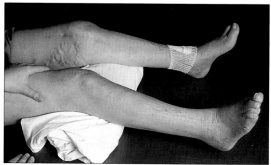

Fig. 7 *Quadriceps wasting. The bulk of the muscle is best felt while the patient tries to extend the knee.*

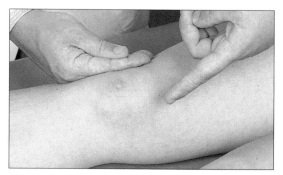

Fig. 8 *The bulge sign for small effusions. Pressure is applied to the lateral side and the examiner looks on the medial side for evidence of a bulge appearing due to fluid flowing across the joint.*

significant problem than a moderate loss of flexion. Intermittent locking suggests a chronic meniscal injury or loose body. Abnormal laxity may result from destruction of cartilage and underlying bone or from disruption of a ligament.

REFERRED PAIN: hip and lumbar spine disorders may present with pain at the knee, with or without pain at the source of the problem. On examination, movement of the knee will be pain-free as long as the hip is held stationary and the back is not stressed.

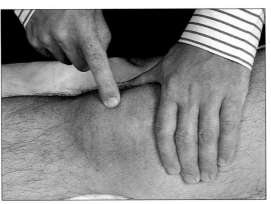

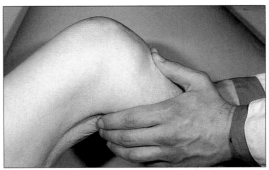

Fig. 11 *Testing stability of cruciate ligaments. The examiner flexes the knee, immobilizes the foot and grasps the upper end of the tibia to see if it will move (rock) forwards and backwards on the femur.*

Fig. 9 *Patellar tap sign for moderate or large effusions. With the supporting hand pressing gently on the suprapatellar pouch to move fluid into the knee joint, the patella is pressed rapidly down against the femoral condyles. When the sign is positive, the patella can be felt to move down 'through' the effusion and knock against the femoral condyles.*

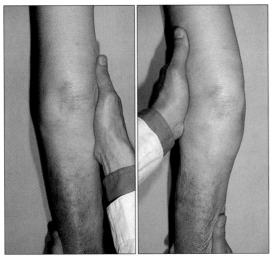

Fig. 10 *Testing stability of collateral ligaments. With the knee slightly flexed, lateral pressure is applied to see if the knee will rock from side to side.*

Not to be Missed

- **Acute infection:** the most important diagnosis to be considered when a patient presents with an acutely painful, swollen knee (see 'The Acutely Painful Joint').
- **Subacute or chronic infection:** should be suspected whenever an undiagnosed inflammatory arthritis involves only one joint (most commonly the knee) or a few joints. The signs of inflammation may be only modest, and special culture techniques and/or synovial biopsy may be required to reach the correct diagnosis. Evidence of multiple joint involvement reduces the likelihood that infection is the cause of the arthritis.
- **Crystal-induced arthritis:** usually presents as an acutely inflamed joint and it is at this stage that a positive diagnosis can be most readily made. See 'The Acutely Painful Joint'.
- **Osteomyelitis and bone tumours:** such as osteogenic sarcoma and osteoid osteoma may present with pain in the region of the knee, and they may produce a sympathetic effusion in the joint.

Investigations and Referral

X-ray will help confirm the presence of osteoarthritis (Fig. 12) but radiological evidence of osteoarthritis does not, of course, exclude the presence of other conditions. Blood tests (full blood count; erythrocyte sedimentation rate, ESR; C-reactive protein, CRP; rheumatoid factor) are useful when abnormal but are rarely diagnostic. A positive rheumatoid factor (low titre) is common in the elderly and does not, in itself, provide evidence of rheumatoid arthritis. Joint aspiration (Fig. 13) and synovial fluid examination is useful when an unexplained monarthritis is present or when infection or crystal induced arthritis (gout or calcium pyrophosphate deposition disease) is suspected.

The knee joint is the commonest site for a wide range of rare disorders; any persistent undiagnosed arthritis or clear mechanical abnormality warrants specialist review.

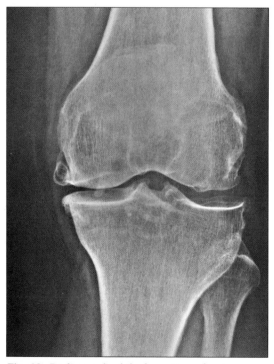

Fig. 12 *Radiograph of the knee in moderate osteoarthritis showing joint space narrowing and sclerosis around the margin of the bone. Characteristic 'tear-drop' osteophytes are also apparent.*

Management

Osteoarthritis

This is the commonest cause of knee pain, and is usually restricted to people older than 40 years unless the joint has been previously traumatized (e.g. meniscectomy). It may affect any or all of the three compartments of the joint (Fig. 14). Stiffness in the morning or after rest is sometimes prominent but short-lived (less than 15 minutes) and systemic markers of inflammation (fatigue, weight loss, ESR, CRP) are absent or normal. On examination the joint is cool with hard swelling, crepitus on movement and sometimes a small effusion. Localized tender spots around the joint line or just below the medial joint line are common (Fig. 15). X-rays of symptomatic joints help to confirm the diagnosis, but the degree of radiological abnormality correlates poorly with the severity of symptoms. Blood tests are only required if other diagnoses, such as rheumatoid arthritis, require exclusion. Management should include education, maintenance of muscle strength by encouraging physical activity and quadriceps exercises, and, when appropriate, advice

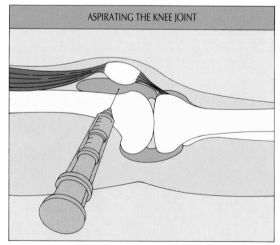

ASPIRATING THE KNEE JOINT

Fig. 13 *Aspirating the knee joint. There are several possible sites of entry; here, with the medial approach, the needle is inserted into the knee joint proper. The patella and femur can be palpated and the needle is inserted into the space beneath the patella at its mid-point. The condylar anatomy is such that the space is wider on the medial side.*

regarding walking sticks and footwear. Drug treatment with analgesics (paracetemol) or non-steroidal anti-inflammatory drugs (usually only required intermittently) is often useful and, for advanced disease, surgery (joint replacement or occasionally, osteotomy) may be indicated.

Traumatic Sequelae

A history of trauma may suggest a meniscal injury, in which case the injury is usually that of a twisting strain on a partially flexed, weight bearing knee resulting in a tear of the medial meniscus. Typically, the knee is painful immediately after the injury and there may be associated locking (inability to extend), and swelling. Chronic meniscal injuries may lead to recurrent pain and locking and subsequently to premature osteoarthritis. The diagnosis may be confirmed by arthrography, arthroscopy or MRI scanning. Rest, splinting, then physiotherapy are sometimes sufficient but more often surgery is required. Trauma may also result in ligamentous injuries, which when complete, result in abnormal movement of the joint and may require surgical repair.

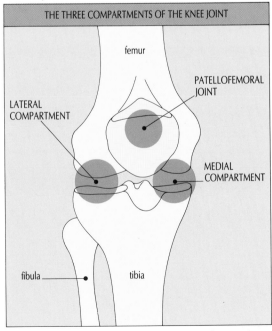

Fig. 14 *The three compartments of the knee joint (right knee, from the front).*

Anterior Knee Pain in Young Adults (Chondromalacia Patellae)

Knee pain in teenage or young women (sometimes men) is often felt anteriorly (behind the patella) and is typically aggravated by sporting activity or negotiating stairs. The knee examination is usually normal apart from pain produced by pressing or rubbing the patella against the underlying femoral condyles (Fig. 16). The association between anterior knee pain and cartilage abnormalities on the undersurface of the patella is weak. A confident diagnosis, reassurance and the avoidance of surgical intervention are the key points in management. Quadriceps exercises are usually helpful.

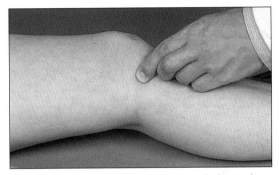

Fig. 15 *Tenderness just below the medial joint line in the region of the insertion of the medial collateral ligament is a common site of 'joint' tenderness, particularly in association with osteoarthritis.*

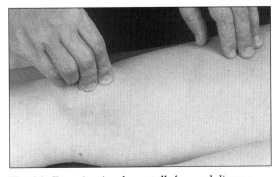

Fig. 16 *Examination for patellofemoral disease. Pressure is being applied to the patella while the patient contracts the quadriceps muscle. The examiner may feel patellofemoral crepitus, and the patient feels pain.*

THE FOOT AND ANKLE

Presentation

Pain and a tendency to 'give way' are the commonest presentations of ankle and foot disorders. Pain in the foot may arise from the forefoot (metatarsalgia), midfoot (tarsal pain) and hindfoot. The majority of disorders giving rise to foot pain are mechanical in origin, resulting from trauma or inappropriate footwear. Arthritis is a less frequent cause of foot and ankle symptoms.

Common Problems

Common causes of foot and ankle pain include:

- **Metatarsalgia (mechanical forefoot pain):** pain occurs in the region of the metatarsal heads, initially on walking but subsequently at rest. This symptom results from any alteration of weight distribution on the foot.
- **Bunion and hallux valgus:** is a very common combination in middle-aged or elderly women (see 'Management', below).
- **Trauma:** an ankle sprain usually follows a forced inversion injury and represents

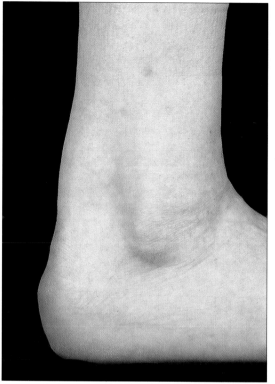

Fig. 1 *Thickening of the Achilles tendon due to repetitive microtrauma associated with sport.*

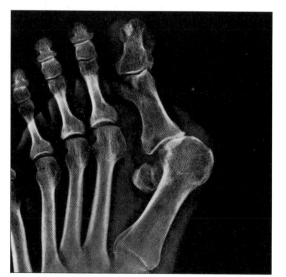

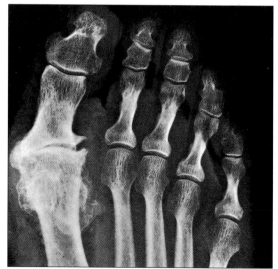

Fig. 2 *Radiological changes of advanced hallux valgus and hallux rigidus. Angulation deformity and subluxation (left) ; bone overgrowth and osteophyte formation immobilizing the joint in hallux rigidus (right).*

damage to the lateral collateral ligament. Sprains recover slowly, and referral is only required if symptoms persist for longer than six months. In middle-aged women, recurrent, minor injury to the lateral ligament may occur in an ankle that 'gives way'. Treatment is physiotherapy to improve muscle-strength and co-ordination.

Rupture of the Achilles tendon occurs usually in middle-age and is often complete. The rupture produces a sharp pain and the patient often feels he has been struck from behind. In younger patients an incomplete rupture near the musculotendinous junction may occur. Careful assessment of the severity of the trauma and its relationship to symptoms is required as patients often relate joint problems to minor trauma inappropriately.

- **Bursitis and peritendonitis:** over-use or friction may produce pain at the back of the heel due to inflammation of the Achilles paratenon or the bursae around the Achilles tendon (Fig. 1).
- **Arthritis:** osteoarthritis most frequently involves the first metatarsophalangeal joint and occurs independently of hallux valgus. A progressive loss of movement may lead to hallux rigidus (Fig. 2).

Rheumatoid and other inflammatory arthritides frequently affect the feet and ankles, but usually in the presence of clear involvement elsewhere.

Seronegative spondyloarthropathies (ankylosing spondylitis, Reiter's disease, etc.) may produce pain in the foot and ankle, due either to arthritis or enthesitis (Achilles tendinitis (Fig. 3), plantar fasciitis). A diffusely swollen ('sausage') toe suggests psoriatic arthritis or Reiter's disease (Fig. 4).

- **Gout:** the joints of the foot and ankle are by far the most commonly involved in gout; the first metatarsophalangeal (MTP) joint is involved in 90% of gout patients at some stage. Abrupt onset and typical distribution (first MTP, tarsal and ankle joints) in a middle-aged man strongly suggest the diagnosis which should, nevertheless, be confirmed whenever possible. See 'The Acutely Painful Joint'.

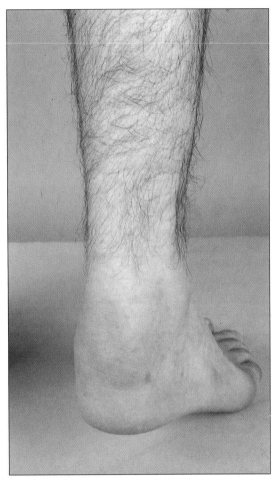

Fig. 3 *Achilles tendonitis in Reiter's disease.*

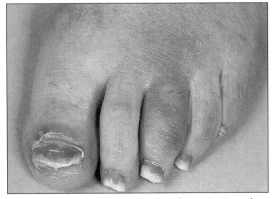

Fig. 4 *Sausage toe associated with psoriatic nail dystrophy. Identical swelling may occur in Reiter's disease.*

Functional Anatomy

Pain in the foot and ankle may arise from the joints and bursae or the tendons, ligaments, fascia and their insertions (Figs 5 & 6). The joints comprise three separate functional groups: the tibiotalar joint which allows plantar and dorsiflexion of the foot, The subtalar joint which allows inversion and eversion, and the midtarsal joints which allow supination and pronation of the forefoot.

Examination

Inspection of the patient's gait, and shoes, is useful (Fig. 7).

LOOK: for deformity of the ankle – best seen from behind, with the patient standing. Note whether the longitudinal arch is preserved and assess the alignment of the forefoot and hindfoot (Fig. 8). The combination of deformity and ill-fitting shoes may lead to callus formation or to ulceration (Fig. 9).

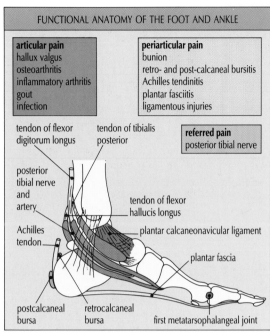

Fig. 6 *Functional anatomy of the foot and ankle.*

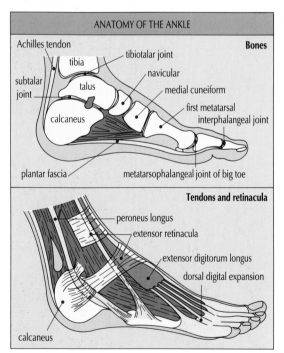

Fig. 5 *Anatomy of the foot and ankle, showing relationship of bones (upper; medial aspect), and tendons and retinacula (lower; lateral aspect).*

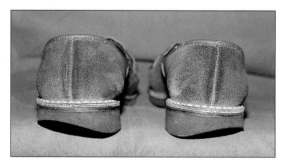

Fig. 7 *Examination of the patient's shoes. This pair shows very uneven heel wear.*

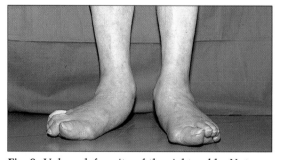

Fig. 8 *Valgus deformity of the right ankle. Note also the loss of the longitudinal arch of the foot.*

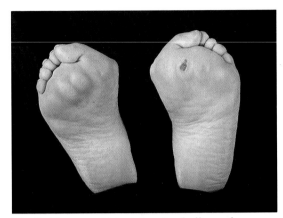

Fig. 9 *Rheumatoid feet showing hallux valgus, MTP subluxation and bursal swellings under the weight-bearing areas. Note the ulcerated area under the left metatarsal heads.*

Swelling may be seen involving tendon sheaths, bursae or joints.

FEEL: for areas of localized tenderness about joints, tendons or fascia (Fig. 10). Pain on lateral compression across the metatarsals is an early sign of inflammation of the MTP joints. Complete rupture of the Achilles tendon is painful and the defect is palpable.

MOVE: to determine the range of motion of the ankle, subtalar and midtarsal joints, and to check for instability (Fig. 11). Pain and deformity are more important causes of functional impairment than loss of movement.

REFERRED PAIN: in the foot may be caused by irritation of the L5–S1 nerve roots by spinal disease (the pain is usually in the lateral half and the sole).

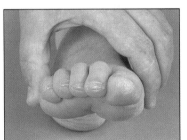
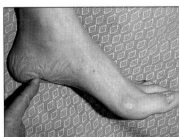
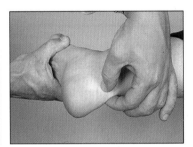

Fig. 10 *Examining for tenderness. Pain on lateral compression across the metatarsals is an early sign of inflammation of the MTP joints (left). Tenderness at the insertion of the plantar fascia into the calcaneum (centre) and of the Achilles tendon (right) is often found in the seronegative spondyloarthropathies.*

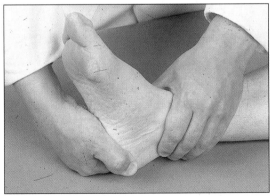
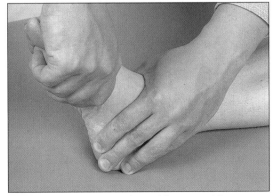

Fig. 11 *The range of movement of the subtalar joint (left) is assessed by fixing the ankle joint with one hand while the calcaneus is rocked from side to side. Midtarsal joint movement (right) is assessed by immobilizing the hindfoot and rotating the forefoot.*

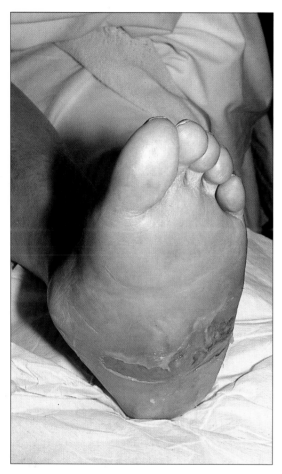

Not to be Missed

- **Diabetic foot:** the combination of neuropathic arthropathy and impaired vascular supply presents a major problem in long-standing diabetes mellitus. Broadening of the midtarsal region and a rocker-bottom foot caused by collapse of the midtarsal structures is characteristic (Fig. 12). Good foot care is essential to prevent the development of skin ulceration and subsequent infection.

Investigations and Referral

Tests are rarely required. X-rays will demonstrate problems of alignment, and they are particularly useful in rheumatoid arthritis as erosions can be detected in the small joints of the feet (even in the absence of foot symptoms) before they are evident elsewhere. Calcaneal spurs (Fig. 13) are very common and usually asymptomatic. X-rays are of much less value in the diagnosis of hindfoot disorders.

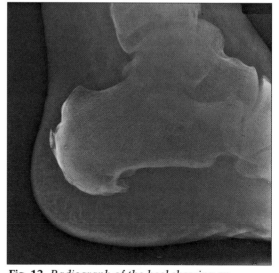

Fig. 12 *Diabetic Charcot joint. There is gross and, initially, relatively painless distortion of the foot anatomy (upper). Pressure has resulted in an ulcer which has become infected. The radiograph shows disruption of intertarsal and tarsometatarsal joints (lower). Note also the arterial calcification indicative of diabetic atherosclerosis.*

Fig. 13 *Radiograph of the heel showing an osteoarthritic calcaneal spur at the insertion of the plantar fascia. These spurs are usually symptomless.*

Blood tests are rarely useful if only the foot is involved. Joint aspiration and synovial fluid examination is useful when infection or crystal-induced arthritis is suspected.

Referral for special footwear or surgery is appropriate when foot pain has not responded to simple measures such as using good supportive shoes (such as lace-up trainers).

Management

Metatarsalgia (Mechanical Forefoot Pain)

The most frequent causes of pain in the region of the metatarsal heads are structural disorders of the whole foot, such as pes planus, and disorders of individual toes, such as hallux valgus and hallux rigidus. Important, though rare, causes include stress fractures of the metatarsals, osteochondritis and Morton's metatarsalgia. The last of these arises from compression of a neuroma on one or more of the plantar digital nerves by the metatarsal heads.

Symptoms may be relieved by shock-absorbing footwear ('trainers'), or metatarsal domes or bars (obtained from shoe shops or chemists). Surgical exploration is only required if a neuroma is suspected and therefore is infrequently performed in metatarsalgia.

Hallux Valgus

Hallux valgus is more frequent among populations that wear shoes and occurs more commonly in women than in men. Although footwear is the most important extrinsic factor there are also intrinsic anatomical factors which predispose to the condition. The valgus deformity tends to increase with age and is frequently associated with thickening and inflammation of the overlying bursa (bunion; Fig. 14).

The condition is potentially preventable by avoiding tight-fitting shoes. Once the deformity has developed, the only options are the use of sufficiently wide shoes to minimize friction, and surgery. Several surgical techniques have been advocated; results are generally good, providing the procedure appropriate for the deformity is adopted. Delayed healing and wound infection are significant problems, however, and the operation should not be considered minor.

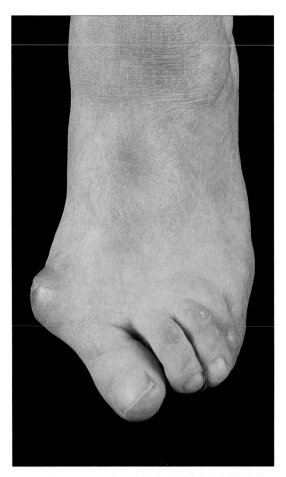

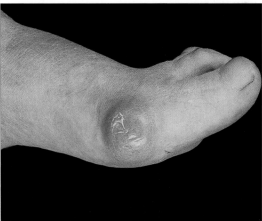

Fig. 14 *Severe hallux valgus with bunion formation. The angulation deformity of the toe is clearly shown (upper) and soft tissue swelling over the bony prominence can be seen (lower).*

3.49

Presentation

Patients of all ages may complain of generalized aches and pains. Pain all over (or more usually pain and stiffness in many sites) may develop suddenly or gradually, or may build up by recruiting sites one at a time over many weeks. For some people, just a few arthritic joints make them feel they have pain everywhere; others will identify more and more sites of complaint the more you show an interest in them. Symptoms are frequently accompanied by lethargy, anxiety or sleep disturbance, and can lead to major loss of function.

Common Problems

- **Depression and anxiety:** even in younger people generalized debility may be a presenting factor. Many patients will readily associate their symptoms with emotional stress.
- **Post-viral syndrome:** lethargy and muscle aches (often in the neck, upper arm and chest wall) in young and middle-aged adults often occur without a clear history of upper respiratory tract infection. There may be a history of increased stress but the patient denies being depressed. The syndrome lasts several weeks or a few months and gradually recovers; investigations, including a virology screen, are negative.
- **Multiple regional pain syndromes:** for example, neck ache, shoulder pain, epicondylitis at the elbow, and carpal tunnel syndrome sometimes occur all at the same time.
- **'Fibromyalgia'** is a poorly defined syndrome of multiple 'trigger points' and limited areas of diffuse tenderness in muscles at sites not related to those of regional pain syndromes. It is sometimes accompanied by lethargy and sleep disturbance.
- **Arthritis:** osteoarthritis, especially in older women, can often affect many sites: pain in fingers, thumb bases, knees and toes may feel like pain all over. Rheumatoid arthritis (RA), particularly affecting fingers, wrists, shoulders, knees and feet, may develop quite rapidly in many joints. There will usually be clear signs of arthritis. In the much less

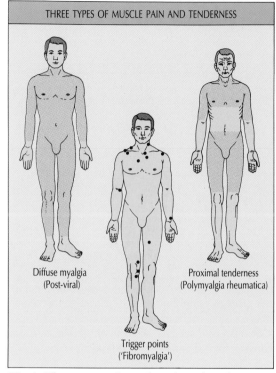

Fig. 1 *Three types of muscle pain and tenderness.*

THREE TYPES OF MUSCLE PAIN AND TENDERNESS

Diffuse myalgia (Post-viral)

Trigger points ('Fibromyalgia')

Proximal tenderness (Polymyalgia rheumatica)

common condition systemic lupus erythematosus, there may be a lot of joint pain (arthralgia) but little sign of arthritis. Ankylosing spondylitis may cause diffuse neck, back and thigh pains, as well as occasional peripheral joint inflammation.
- **Polymyalgia rheumatica (PMR).** Pain and stiffness occurs in the proximal muscles (Fig. 1). Marked early morning stiffness in the shoulder and hip girdle, sometimes making it very difficult to get out of bed or even turn over in bed, is the hallmark, and it may be accompanied by general malaise and weight loss. It rarely occurs in people under 60.

Functional Anatomy

Somatic complaints can be induced by anxiety and depression, so the identification of specific sites of pain and tenderness does not exclude these diagnoses.

Regional pain syndrome lesions occur at ligaments, tendons and bursae (Fig. 2). 'Trigger points' are small areas (about 1 cm across) of intense muscle

SITES OF SYMPTOMS IN 'PAIN ALL OVER'			
	Pain	Stiffness	Tenderness
Joints	●	●	●
Ligament and tendon insertions	●		●
Bones	●		●
Muscles – radiation	●		●
Muscles – general	●	●	●
Muscles – specific points			●
Nerves	●		
Bursae	●		●

Fig. 2 *Sites of symptoms in 'pain all over'.*

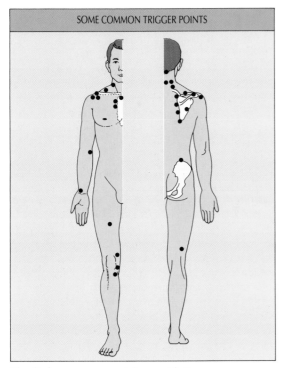

SOME COMMON TRIGGER POINTS

Fig. 3 *Some common trigger points.*

tenderness, often surrounded by areas of muscle spasm. They occur in many areas but frequently follow a well recognized pattern (Fig. 3) and pain may radiate diffusely into the surrounding areas. The site of the symptoms may not be the site of the pathology, just as pain may radiate to a distant site. The features of arthritis are dealt with in other chapters. Proximal muscle tenderness usually occurs in the neck, shoulders and upper arms, and in the buttocks and thighs.

Not to be Missed

- **A new problem in patients with long-standing aches and pains.** Osteoarthritis of many joints is common in the elderly, but does not prevent the development of PMR or RA.

- **Temporal arteritis** (Fig. 4) may present with a similar picture to polymyalgia rheumatica (with which it overlaps) but be accompanied by headaches, temporal artery tenderness, and sometimes visual disturbances (Fig. 5).

- **Systemic diseases,** including hypothyroidism, diabetes, Paget's disease, peripheral neuropathy and vitamin D deficiency (osteomalacia), sometimes produce complaints of diffuse, difficult to describe symptoms. Neoplasia, particularly multiple myeloma but also multiple secondary deposits from almost any primary tumour, can cause similar problems.

- **Myositis,** inflammation in muscles, is a rare condition of middle-aged adults and is occasionally seen in children. Proximal muscle weakness is the key feature. Ask the patient to squat and rise unaided or raise arms against resistance to test for this. Most patients also develop an erythematous rash and some have general malaise. Serum creatinine phosphokinase (CPK) levels are raised and urgent specialist treatment is required.

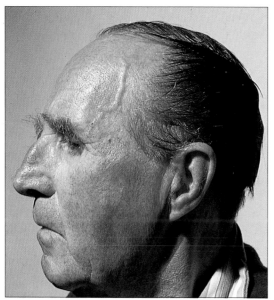

Fig. 4 *Prominent left temporal artery in a patient with giant cell arteritis. The artery was tender and non-pulsatile.*

RELATIONSHIP BETWEEN POLYMYALGIA RHEUMATICA AND TEMPORAL ARTERITIS	
TA Cranial artery tenderness, swelling and loss of pulse Headache Jaw claudication Visual disturbances 50% female	**Acute phase response** Malaise Fatigue Depression Weight loss Fever
PMR and TA	
PMR Proximal muscle pain Early morning stiffness Prompt, dramatic response to low doses of steroid 85% female	

Fig. 5 *Differences, similarities and overlap between polymyalgia rheumatica and temporal arteritis: 60% of patients have PMR, 20% TA, and 20% both.*

Examination

The main purpose of the examination will be to establish the site and nature of any focal lesions. A common differential diagnosis is shoulder capsulitis, PMR and RA (Fig. 6).

LOOK: for signs of arthritis and the distribution of joints involved.

FEEL: for localized areas of tenderness. Characterize each lesion to see if it relates to a bursa, tendon, ligament or joint.

MOVE: to test joint range — restriction suggests arthritis. Test muscle strength remembering that full strength may be held only momentarily due to pain at joints or ligaments. True muscle weakness is an unusual, sinister component of pain all over, suggesting severe disease (myopathy, myositis, neoplasia).

Investigation and Referral

An elevated acute phase response (ESR, plasma viscosity, C-reactive protein) usually indicates an underlying inflammatory condition. These may also cause a small rise in alkaline phosphatase, but higher levels with a normal ESR suggest metabolic bone disease. Referral may be worthwhile if any of these abnormalities emerge, and for psychogenic symptoms if simple management proves ineffective.

Management
Multiple Regional Pain Syndromes

Each of these should be treated separately. Local heat treatment followed by exercises is often helpful, and for specific lesions, steroid and/or local anaesthetic injections may prove helpful. Strong reassurance that the patient does not have a generalized systemic disease is usually worthwhile. Analgesics and anti-inflammatory agents usually make little contribution to symptom control. For resistant lesions physiotherapy may help.

'Fibromyalgia'

Individual or particularly troublesome trigger points

A COMMON DIAGNOSTIC PROBLEM AT THE SHOULDER			
	Capsulitis	*Rheumatoid arthritis*	*Polymyalgia rheumatica*
Pain	Around shoulder	In shoulder	Across neck and shoulder muscles
	May radiate diffusely into biceps and triceps	On moving joint	In upper arm muscles
	On stressing capsule or ligaments		
Stiffness	On waking	On waking	Severe on waking
	Persistent	After rest	May resolve during day
	Near joint	In the joint	In neck, shoulder and upper arm
Tenderness	At specific sites	In joint line	In muscles
Restriction of movement	In relation to specific tendons	Generalized	None or little
Concomitant features	May be a history of waxing and waning and differential development in the two shoulders	Usually a peripheral symmetrical polyarthritis	Usually similar symptoms in pelvic girdle

Fig. 6 *A common diagnostic problem at the shoulder.*

may be treated with local heat, rubifacients and massage, or occasionally local infiltration of steroids. Sleep disturbance and depression may contribute to the development of lesions and be induced by them. Amitriptyline 25–75 mg at night for 3–6 months may be beneficial. Relaxation techniques help some patients, and some community psychiatric nurses are prepared to help in management.

Arthritis

See the appropriate management section in this book.

Polymyalgia Rheumatica

It is easy to have too low a threshold for diagnosing this condition (especially to confuse it with bilateral soft tissue lesions of the shoulders), to be over aggressive with early treatment and to reduce treatment too soon. Clear-cut cases will be over 60 years of age, have an elevated acute phase response (e.g. ESR) and will markedly respond (clinically and ESR) within 48 hours to 15 mg prednisolone daily, the symptoms quickly re-appearing on stopping the steroids one week later. Occasionally rheumatoid arthritis or other systemic diseases present in a similar way to polymyalgia rheumatica. It is almost certainly worth referring patients suspected of having polymyalgia, but in whom these criteria are not met, for a specialist opinion *before* starting longer term steroid therapy. Once the diagnosis is established an acceptable treatment regimen might be 15 mg prednisolone daily for 4 weeks, 12.5 mg daily for 4–6 weeks, 10 mg daily for 8–12 months, then slowly reduce the steroid level by 1 mg/month over the following year. A few patients will have a recrudescence of their symptoms requiring a restart of this treatment schedule, and some will never be able to completely stop their steroid treatment because of the development of aches and pains whenever they go below, say, 5 mg/day.

Section 4

NON-REGIONAL PRESENTATIONS

A PAINFUL RED EYE may be the presentation of a reactive arthritis (conjunctivitis), and can occur in ankylosing spondylitis (uveitis) and rheumatoid arthritis (scleritis).

DRY, 'GRITTY' EYES may develop in patients with or without arthritis, due to Sjögren's syndrome.

- **Reiter's disease:** occurs mostly in young men. The classical triad is conjunctivitis, urethritis and a predominantly lower-limb arthritis. Mouth ulcers, circinate balinitis and keratodermia blenorrhagica can also occur. Various combinations of two or more of these features may be present (Fig. 1).

- **Ankylosing spondylitis:** is another disease of young men. Preceding or intercurrent attacks of uveitis may be the clue to the diagnosis of a young person with back or limb pains (Fig. 2).

- **Sjögren's syndrome:** occurs mostly in middle aged women, with or without rheumatoid arthritis or another rheumatic disease. Dry eyes and mouth, lacrymal and salivary gland swelling, dryness of the vagina, malaise, and aches and pains, often occur (Fig. 3). Artificial tears are needed to protect the eyes from scarring.

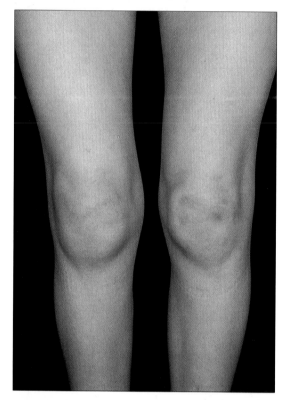

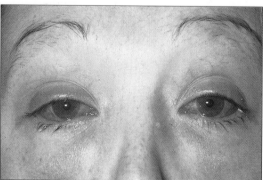

Fig. 1 *Synovitis of the knee (upper) and conjunctivitis (lower) in Reiter's syndrome. Courtesy of Professor H. Lambert.*

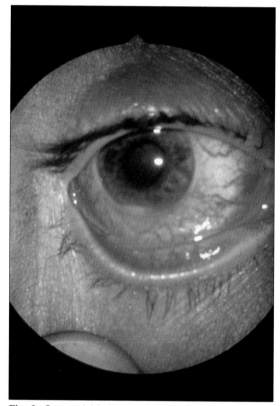

Fig. 2 *Severe iritis in a patient with ankylosing spondylitis, showing considerable conjunctival infection and a hypopyon.*

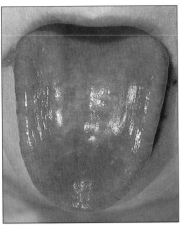
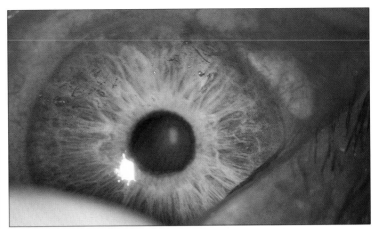

Fig. 3 *Sjögren's syndrome: dry tongue with mucosal atrophy (left) and dry eyes with keratitis demonstrated by Rose Bengal staining (right; courtesy of Mr Paul A. Hunter).*

Not to be Missed

- **Uveitis in children:** some children with arthritis develop symptomless uveitis with damage to their sight (Fig. 4). They may need regular ophthalmological screening.

- **Scleromalacia perforans and corneal melt:** severe rheumatoid arthritis with scleritis sometimes results in perforation of the anterior chamber of the eye (Fig. 5).

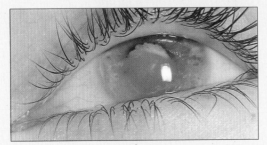

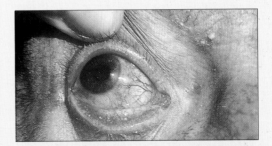

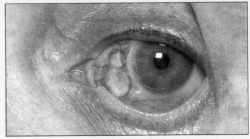

Fig. 4 *Uveitis in children. Early stage: anterior chamber clouding (upper). Late chronic stage: scarring, and secondary cataract (lower).*

Fig. 5 *Severe episcleritis in a patient with RA (upper). Eye disease in RA occasionally leads to perforation of the anterior chamber (lower).*

Most of the diseases which produce a skin rash and arthritis will fall into one of the five main groups listed in Fig. 1.

CAUSES OF ARTHRITIS AND SKIN RASH
Psoriasis, Reiter's disease
Systemic lupus erythematosus and its variants Dermatomyositis Juvenile chronic arthritis

Vasculitis
    rheumatoid arthritis
    polyarteritis nodosa
    Henoch–Schönlein purpura
    cryoglobulinaemia
    erythema nodosum

Infections
    viral
    spirochaetal
    gonococcal and meningococcal

Drugs

Fig. 1 *Causes of arthritis and a skin rash.*

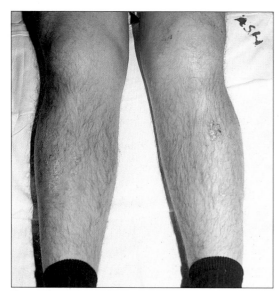

Fig. 2 *Psoriatic arthritis. Note the right knee effusion and psoriatic patches on the shins.*

• **Psoriasis** may be associated with several different patterns of inflammatory arthritis (Fig. 2). Peripheral joints are usually involved but axial involvement of the 'ankylosing spondylitis' type may also occur. Reiter's disease produces a rash on the soles of the feet which closely resembles pustular psoriasis.

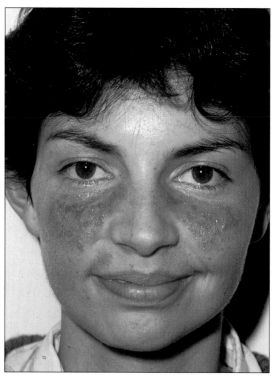

Fig. 3 *Butterfly rash of systemic lupus erythematosus.*

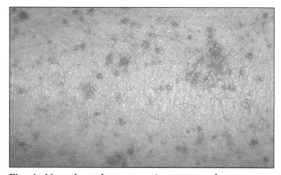

Fig. 4 *Non-thrombocytopenic purpura due to leucocytoclastic vasculitis.*

- **Systemic lupus erythematosus** and its variants frequently produce a skin rash in association with a non-erosive symmetrical, usually mild, polyarthritis. Several different types of rash may occur, but most characteristic are the butterfly (Fig. 3) and diffuse erythematous rashes of systemic lupus erythematosus.

- **Vasculitis involving small vessels** (capillaries, arterioles, venules) typically produces non-thrombocytopenic purpura, a rash which is palpable and sometimes tender (neither of which is true of thrombocytopenic purpura) (Fig. 4). Histology of the rash shows a leucocytoclastic vasculitis but is not specific for the underlying disease. Of the many causes, rheumatoid arthritis, Henoch–Schönlein purpura, Wegener's granulomatosis or drugs are the most common in patients with a concomitant arthritis. In rheumatoid arthritis, small-vessel occlusion may also produce nail-edge infarcts which are sometimes associated with systemic vasculitis (Fig. 5).

- **Erythema nodosum** (Fig. 6), a type of paniculitis, is frequently associated with an arthritis/periarthritis, most commonly involving the ankles.

- **Viral and bacterial infections** may produce arthritis and a rash, although most commonly rubella or hepatitis B is responsible.

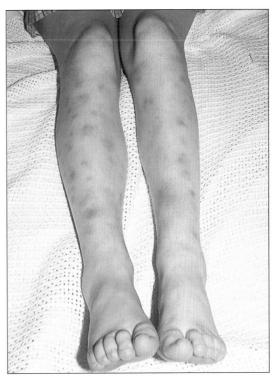

Fig. 6 *Erythema nodosum in a patient with acute sarcoidosis.*

Not to be Missed

- **Skin necrosis due to necrotizing arteritis** (Fig. 7) signals the presence of severe systemic vasculitis and the need for urgent referral.

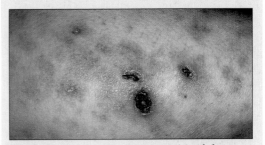

Fig. 7 *Systemic necrotizing arteritis of the polyarteritis nodosa type, producing necrotic patches due to small arterial involvement. The same may occur in rheumatoid arthritis.*

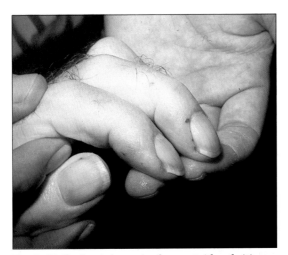

Fig. 5 *Nail-edge infarcts in rheumatoid arthritis indicate small vessel occlusion and are sometimes associated with systemic vasculitis.*

Arthritis is often accompanied by lumps and bumps, although the latter are rarely a presenting feature or a symptomatic problem.

SOFT SWELLING AROUND THE JOINTS may be due to bursitis, tenosynovitis or synovial extensions of joints (Fig. 1). They are often painful or tender on pressure and movement. They indicate an inflammatory arthritis.

FIRM SUBCUTANEOUS LUMPS often develop on the elbows, hands, Achilles tendon and other pressure areas (Fig. 1). Rheumatoid nodules, gouty tophi and xanthomata are the commoner causes. Nodules occasionally develop in other inflammatory disorders such as SLE and rheumatic fever.

- **The rheumatoid nodule:** look carefully at the hands and feel along the ulnar border of the forearm and the Achilles tendon. Rheumatoid nodules vary in size enormously (Fig. 2). They are usually firm, non-tender swellings attached to tendon or periosteum, but not to skin. They occasionally precede arthritis, but more usually develop in established, sero-positive disease (about thirty per cent of rheumatoid sufferers get nodules). Nodules on the Achilles tendon can cause problems with shoes (Fig. 3), and elsewhere they may cause

mechanical problems, and ulcers. They are unsightly.

- **Heberden's nodes:** firm swellings either side of the distal or proximal interphalangeal joints develop in osteoarthritis of the hand (Fig. 4). They often go through phases of irritation and tender-

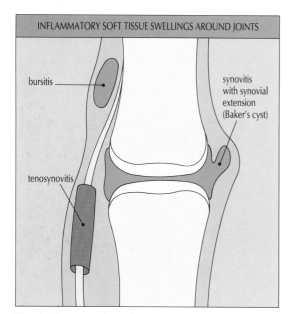

Fig. 1 *Patterns of swelling around the joints.*

INFLAMMATORY SOFT TISSUE SWELLINGS AROUND JOINTS

bursitis

synovitis with synovial extension (Baker's cyst)

tenosynovitis

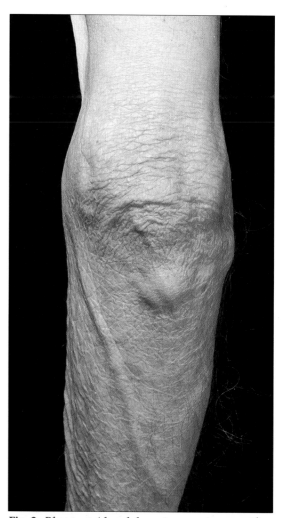

Fig. 2 *Rheumatoid nodules occur most commonly on the extensor surface of the forearm, just below the olecranon process. They may be attached to periosteum but not to skin. They are not usually tender. As they may be very small and go unnoticed by the patient, careful palpation along the ulnar border may be necessary to detect this important physical sign.*

ness, but usually settle after a few years, leaving painless, swollen, stiff joints. Their presence may be a clue to the diagnosis of osteoarthritis elsewhere (such as the knees). They should not be confused with asymptomatic fibro-fatty pads over the knuckles, which have no significance (Garrod's fatty pads).

Not to be Missed

- **The sacral nodule:** may ulcerate in immobile rheumatoid sufferers with disastrous results (Fig. 5). Look out for sacral nodules and others on pressure areas, and attend to skin care and pressure relief.

- **The gouty tophus:** elderly women on diuretics sometimes develop gouty tophi on the hands and feet, without any gouty arthritis. The lesions can be mistaken for septic arthritis or other problems (Fig. 6).

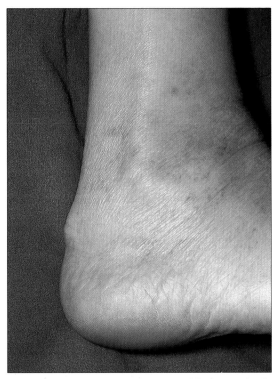

Fig. 3 *Rheumatoid nodule on the Achilles tendon.*

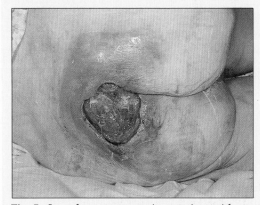

Fig. 5 *Sacral pressure sore in a patient with longstanding rheumatoid arthritis.*

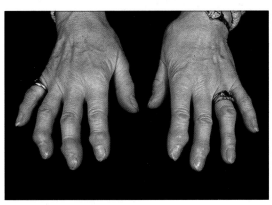

Fig. 4 *Heberden's nodes.*

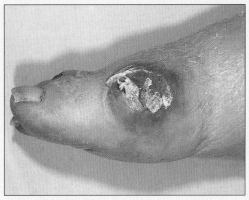

Fig. 6 *Gouty tophus.*

Fever and malaise are systemic consequences of inflammation. They may be due to the cause of a rheumatic disease, or be the result of an inflammatory arthritis.

- **Viral infections** may produce fever, malaise and polyarthritis, often in association with a rash (Fig. 1). The commonest cause is rubella (Fig. 2), but

INFECTIONS PRODUCING FEVER, MALAISE AND POLYARTHRITIS	
Viruses	rubella
	hepatitis B
	parvovirus
	arboviruses (Africa, Australia)
Bacteria	gonococcus, meningococcus
	Lyme disease
Reactive	post-streptococcal (rheumatic fever)

Fig. 1 *Infections that frequently produce fever, malaise and polyarthritis.*

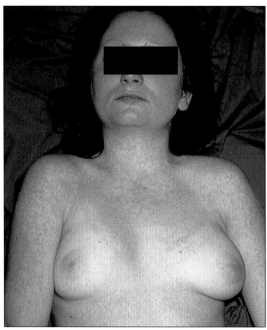

Fig. 2 *The characteristic rash of rubella. Courtesy of Professor H. Lambert.*

parvovirus ('slapped cheek' or 'fifth disease') can also cause outbreaks affecting many people. The prodromal phases of hepatitis may include polyarthritis, and polyarthralgia or myalgia can accompany many other infections, including influenza. Bacterial and other organisms can also cause febrile illnesses with malaise and arthritis; gonorrhoea is particularly likely to result in upper limb arthritis, with or without tenosynovitis, and can cause diagnostic confusion.

- **Active arthritis** with a lot of local inflammation will cause systemic symptoms such as malaise. Sometimes there is a mild fever, with night sweats (Fig. 3). However, the sudden development of systemic features, and high fevers, should always prompt a careful examination for *sepsis*. Patients with chronic arthritis are prone to joint infections, but they can obviously develop a variety of other infectious diseases as well.

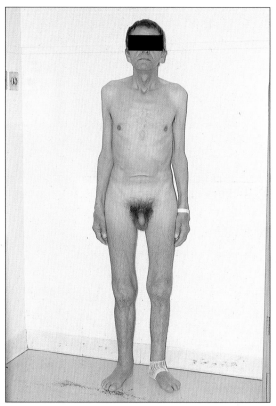

Fig. 3 *Weight loss, malaise and low grade fever reflect active disease in rheumatoid arthritis.*

Not to be Missed

- **Malignancy:** malignant disease can result in systemic symptoms, as well as joint or muscle pains, sometimes accompanied by a fever. Bronchial carcinoma can present with shoulder pains, and it is also the commonest cause of 'HPOA' (Fig. 4). This rare condition causes wrist and ankle pains, with periostitis and clubbing. Local malignant deposits can also present with regional bone, muscle or joint pains, simulating a rheumatic condition.

- **Specific rheumatic conditions:** a variety of the less common rheumatic diseases can cause arthritis with a high fever. Sometimes the febrile illness dominates the condition, and the joint symptoms are either mild or absent.

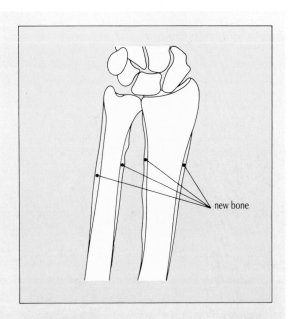

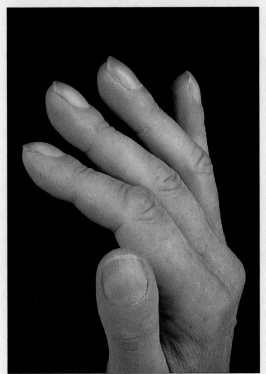

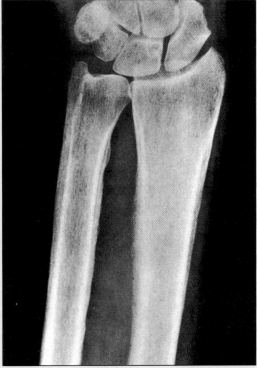

Fig. 4 *Hypertrophic osteoarthropathy produces pain and tenderness of the distal forearm and wrist. The patient is clubbed and the X-ray shows periosteal new bone formation. The cause is usually bronchogenic carcinoma of the lung.*

Systemic onset juvenile chronic arthritis (Still's disease) causes high swinging fevers (Fig. 5), and some of the connective tissue disorders, such as SLE, and polyarteritis and other vasculitides can present in this way. Less commonly, rheumatoid arthritis, ankylosing spondylitis, polyarticular gout, giant cell arteritis and other arthropathies present similarly.

- **Septic arthritis:** primary infections of synovial joints are rare and occur particularly in ill or immunosuppressed patients, and in those with a pre-existing arthritis (Fig. 6). The disc spaces of the spine, as well as synovial joints, can be affected.

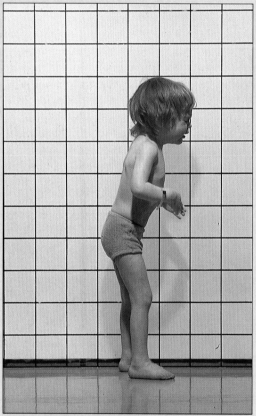

Fig. 5 *A sick child with arthritis and fever may have Still's disease (systemic onset juvenile chronic arthritis).*

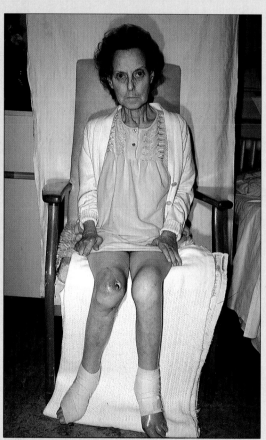

Fig. 6 *Infection of synovial joints in a patient with severe rheumatoid arthritis. Infection from ulcerated skin over the ankles has spread to the knee where the metal prosthesis can be seen at the base of a deep infected ulcer.*

Section 5

APPROACHES TO MANAGEMENT

EDUCATION IN ARTHRITIS

The Problem

- Arthritis is often a chronic disease to which patients must adapt.
- Many patients do not understand the medical model of illness which doctors take for granted.
- Patients and their relatives need to know more about arthritis, its prognosis and its treatment.

Why Intervene?

- Patients want to know about their illness.
- Their use of and benefits from treatment are improved.
- The use of medical resources is reduced.
- Patients take greater responsibility for themselves.
- Patients and relatives can adapt their life to the arthritis.

What is There?

Simple, jargon-free descriptions provided by the patient's doctor or therapist.
Drawings, sketches or pictures for the patient to take away.
Books from the library.
Attractive booklets produced by the Arthritis and Rheumatism Council and the Arthritis Foundation (Fig. 1).
Leaflets from the ARC, pharmaceutical companies, etc., with illustrations and basic advice.
Package inserts with medications.

Example

Anne Jones was an active working wife when she developed rheumatoid arthritis at the age of 26. Inflammation in several fingers and both wrists was bad enough for her to consult her GP. She tried intermittent analgesics and took anti-inflammatory tablets when the pain and stiffness were particularly bad, but mostly she tried to ignore the symptoms in her hands. Eventually she returned to her GP because lack of sleep was making her irritable and preventing her from concentrating at work. She would lie awake at night worrying that she would soon be in a wheel-chair like her elderly aunt.

It took several simple explanations and the opportunity to read a booklet on RA, but Anne gradually understood that although RA was a common disease most patients never became as disabled as her aunt. She accepted that the symptoms varied from day to day, and that regular evening treatment with an anti-inflammatory tablet would help her morning stiffness. On bad mornings she could spend a few minutes with her hands in warm water.

Subsequently her joint symptoms were a little better controlled, but more importantly she seemed more relaxed in her acceptance of her arthritis. She went to work 20 minutes later than previously, to give her a little more time in the mornings. On her next visit to the surgery she was clearly more positive about the future and asked if her arthritis might be affected by having children.

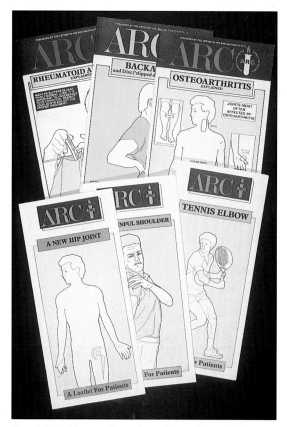

Fig. 1 *Booklets such as these from the ARC are available from a number of organizations.*

Some information helpful to patients with rheumatoid arthritis

- Most patients can cope with their rheumatoid arthritis, and few end up in a wheelchair.

- RA is a very variable condition — it can change from week to week or even from day to day. It can go through periods of remission as well as 'flares' of activity.

- We do not know the cause of RA, nor do we have a cure, but we understand some things about it and can help to improve symptoms and get round problems.

- Tablets to treat RA are either painkillers, anti-inflammatory tablets or tablets which cut down the overall level of arthritis after being taken for several weeks or months. The best combination of treatment for you should be worked out with your doctor.

- When joints are inflamed there are other simple ways of easing symptoms, such as relaxation and the use of heat and cold.

- Exercises can be helpful in keeping the joints mobile and the muscles strong.

- Arthritis is usually worse in the morning and can use up your energy — you can organize your activities to take this into account.

REST AND EXERCISE IN ARTHRITIS

The Problem

- Some patients make their arthritis worse by never giving their joints a rest.
- Others do the opposite, and never achieve their optimum function or symptom control.
- Many are confused as to when exercise and rest are most appropriate.

Why Intervene?

- Both rest and exercise have an important role in controlling symptoms and improving function.
- With help, patients can learn to incorporate their activities into their daily life, so making the best of their abilities.
- Used in the wrong way, exercises could make the problems worse rather than better.

What is There?

Information booklets on arthritis from the ARC, the Arthritis Foundation, etc.
Advice from specialist occupational (remedial) therapists (OTs) and physiotherapists.

Example

Mrs McGregor was determined to be the master of her arthritis, just as she kept control of her psoriasis. Over two years her joint problems had mostly been confined to one finger and her knees, but she then had a more generalized 'flare' involving many joints and making her feel miserable. She redoubled her efforts at exercising and arranged to host the next church coffee morning, just to prove she could cope. Her daughter came to the rescue and insisted that Mrs McGregor see her GP, who asked the OT to call. Mrs McGregor had not understood that she should rest her joints when they were inflamed, and ease off activities on mornings when she was stiff. She learned how to use a relaxation tape and changed the next coffee morning to afternoon tea.

5.3

EXERCISE FOR MUSCLE STRENGTH

The Problem

- Patients with painful joints do not exercise their muscles.
- Muscle wasting can occur rapidly, especially at the knee.
- Weak muscles reduce function, increase fatigue and reduce joint stability, all of which lead to worse symptoms.

Why Intervene?

- Exercise is an important part of the treatment of patients with arthritis.
- Exercises reduce pain, prevent joint deformities, increase strength and generally help patients to perform daily activities more easily.
- Regular exercise can only be achieved by the patient at home and requires repeated encouragement.

What is There?

Exercise: most physiotherapy departments will be happy to teach patients appropriate exercises — this will usually require only a few visits.

Simple leaflets can explain the role of exercise and provide examples.

Repeated encouragement from all concerned will help the patient to maintain commitment.

Example

Miss Pritchard, previously a keen horsewoman but now at 58 a couple of stone overweight and an active member of the club committee, began to develop osteoarthritis of her knees. The pain was particularly severe on rising from a chair or going up and down the stairs, which was troublesome because the clubroom was above the stables. She took less exercise, became more overweight and had even more trouble with her knees, which made her frustrated and upset. Painkillers did not seem to help much. Her GP noticed that her quadriceps muscles had become quite weak and that her main knee pain was coming from the patello-femoral compartments. He asked the physiotherapist attached to his practice to treat Miss Pritchard, and she concentrated particularly on quadriceps strengthening exercises (Fig. 2). It took two or three weeks before any noticeable improvement occurred, and during that time Miss Pritchard had to take paracetamol half an hour before her exercises so that her knees did not hurt too much. Gradually she found this was unnecessary and she was able to be more active with less knee pain. She resolved to do something about her weight in a further effort to reduce symptoms.

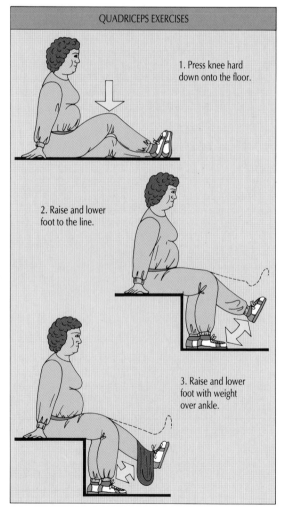

Fig. 2 *Quadriceps exercises.*

EXERCISE FOR JOINT MOBILITY

The Problem

- Joint pain inhibits movement.
- Arthritis and periarthritis can induce joint capsule fibrosis and restriction.
- Flexion deformities and permanent loss of joint range can persist even after inflammation has settled.

Why Intervene?

- Normal function requires adequate joint mobility.
- Exercises can increase joint range and reduce pain.
- Maintaining joint mobility during episodes of arthritis or periarthritis prevents permanent loss of joint mobility after the inflammation has settled.

What is There?

Exercises: most physiotherapy departments will be happy to teach patients appropriate exercises — this will usually require only a few visits.
Simple leaflets can explain the role of exercise and provide examples.
Repeated encouragement from all concerned will help the patient to maintain commitment.

Example

Bill was a Professor of History who fell while at an archaeological dig and hurt his shoulder. Over the next few days the pain seemed to settle into the upper outer arm, was worse at night, and stopped him lying on his left side because of pain at the shoulder tip. Shoulder movements were becoming restricted and he had moved his telephone closer to him because he could not reach out to it across the desk. It was clear that he had developed a capsulitis of his shoulder and although an intra-articular steroid injection relieved the pain and improved his sleep, shoulder movements were, if anything, deteriorating. He saw the physiotherapist three times a week for four weeks, then weekly for another four. She taught him exercises to increase the range of shoulder movement (Fig. 3) and encouraged him to do them every day. By eight weeks he had recovered 80% of shoulder movement and had put his telephone back where it belonged.

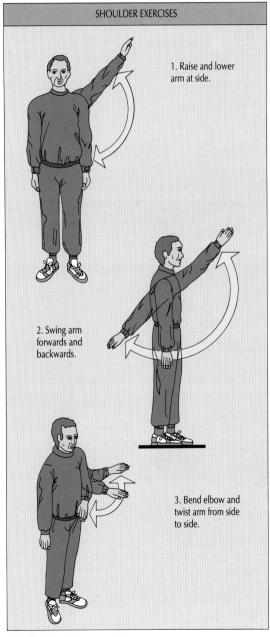

SHOULDER EXERCISES

1. Raise and lower arm at side.

2. Swing arm forwards and backwards.

3. Bend elbow and twist arm from side to side.

Fig. 3 *Shoulder exercises.*

LOCAL TREATMENT OF INFLAMMATION

The Problem

- Inflammation at well-localized sites in the musculo-skeletal system may be difficult to manage with systemic therapy alone.
- Well-localized inflammation may occur as part of a generalized rheumatological disorder such as rheumatoid arthritis, or arise in periarticular soft tissue, often as a result of trauma or unusually energetic use, such as rotator cuff tendonitis.

Why Intervene?

When nonsteroidal anti-inflammatory drugs and rest fail to alleviate the symptoms and signs of inflammation at particular musculoskeletal sites, additional local measures may be useful.

What is There?

Heat (warm soak, electric heat pad, electric lamp, hot water bottle, gel pack; see Fig. 4) is useful for joint pain and stiffness early in the morning or after rest.
Cold (cold water soak, ice/gel pack) is best used for acutely inflamed (hot and swollen) joints.
Ultrasound, short-wave diathermy and transcutaneous nerve stimulation (Fig. 5) are obtainable through a physiotherapy department, and may be useful for soft tissue disorders and more intractable pain.

Example

Hazel is a 50 year old school teacher who has recently developed rheumatoid arthritis. She was started on a nonsteroidal anti-inflammatory drug, which markedly improved her early morning stiffness and the pain in her peripheral joints. She confessed, however, that she still suffered considerable pain in one of her ankles, which was swollen and moderately tender.

The persisting synovitis in Hazel's ankle benefits from local treatment, particularly the application of heat and cold. When the joint was very inflamed, cold was particularly useful. It was applied for about 10 minutes at a time, followed by rest until the numbness wore away. Now that the acute inflammation has subsided, local heat is more effective in reducing pain for short periods, permitting exercises to be done and improving sleep.

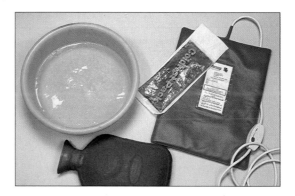

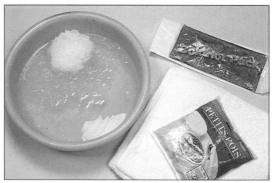

Fig. 4 *Application of heat or cold may be useful at local painful or inflamed sites.*

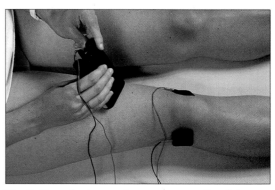

Fig. 5 *Use of a transcutaneous nerve stimulator.*

SPLINTS AND ORTHOSES

The Problem

- A joint may need to be temporarily immobilized to allow an episode of acute inflammation to settle.
- Joint movement may cause pain that can be relieved by support or splinting.
- Joints may become unstable, limiting function and causing pain.

Why Intervene?

- If temporary immobilization of a joint is necessary, application of a splint is the obvious answer.
- There are two other possible objectives — relief of pain and inflammation, and/or improving function.
- In many chronic situations, a well applied splint or orthosis may result in both relief of pain and an improvement in function, without exposing the patient to more hazardous treatments.
- Only when both the prescriber and the patient can see a clear, simple objective and potential 'gain' from the use of an external appliance should one be prescribed.

What is There?

A splint is an external device designed to immobilize part of the body.
An orthosis is used to improve stability and/or reduce pain, while still allowing some movement.

The success of splints and orthoses depends in a large part on the skills of the prescriber, the makers and fitters. Examples include collars and corsets, tennis elbow braces (see 'The Elbow'), wrist and hand splints, knee orthoses, calipers, ankle foot orthoses ('AFOs') and adaptations to footwear (p.5.10). A simple wrist splint often relieves pain and improves grip (Fig. 6); it is an example of a useful aid, freely available 'across the counter' in many shops and in hospital casualty or out-patient departments.

Collars and corsets are probably over-used; most other splints and orthoses are often under-used, or made, fitted and used badly.

Example

May is a 64-year-old lady with rheumatoid arthritis. When she first developed the disease (age 39), many of her joints became very painful, hot and swollen. She was in hospital for a while, where, amongst other things, she had resting wrist splints fitted. These helped the local inflammation settle, and relieved her carpal tunnel symptoms; she went on using them from time to time, whenever the disease 'flared up'. She was also given some knee splints to

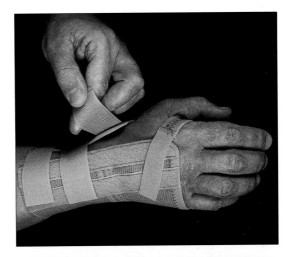

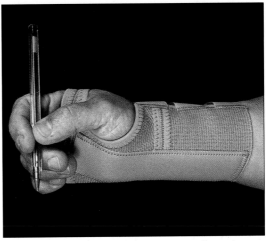

Fig. 6 *A working wrist splint supports the wrist and allows the fingers to move freely, thus improving grip and reducing pain. It can easily be put on and taken off with the help of Velcro fastenings.*

use at night. These helped the knee inflammation, and prevented her from developing flexion deformities (Fig. 7).

Over the last few years the disease has been less active, but it has caused damage to a number of joints. May now finds that wrist splints help relieve pain when she is doing things with her hands, and allow her to grip things better. She now has a collar, which she wears for car journeys or when the pain gets particularly bad. It relieves her neck pain, and gives her a feeling of security when she is travelling. She also uses a small 'AFO', which fits in her right shoe and supports the back of the calf in an unobtrusive fashion. It reduces the valgus deformity of the hind foot, and makes walking easier and less painful.

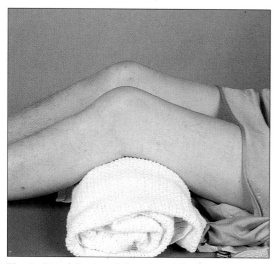

Fig. 7 *Fixed flexion deformity of the knees. Patients with rheumatoid arthritis often find they are more comfortable if the knees are left flexed, and so they sleep with the knees supported on a pillow or rolled-up blankets, as shown here. This encourages the development of a fixed flexion deformity (here about 40°).*

ADL: AIDS TO DAILY LIVING

The Problem

- Arthritis often results in functional problems, disability and handicap (Fig. 8).
- It may be impossible to reverse the process or alter the functional losses resulting from arthritis.

Why Intervene?

- Education can help people overcome disability by showing them ways of doing things in spite of the functional problems.
- Aids and appliances can alter the impact of a functional problem, reducing the disability and handicap.
- Altering the living environment of severely disabled people can enable them to continue independent lives.

What is There?

There are three types of 'aids to daily living':

'Trick' techniques for doing things, and simple 'common-sense' ways of getting round a problem often allow people to manage in spite of a functional problem. Occupational (remedial) therapists (OTs) and fellow sufferers, as well as doctors and other paramedicals, should be available to offer advice and help. There is often a great educational need by the disabled, and what seems obvious to the professionals may be a revelation to the patients.

A variety of 'aids and appliances' are available to help people with simple everyday tasks made impossible by arthritis. The cheap, simple devices are often the most important (Fig. 9). Examples include the dressing stick and tap turner. Handles on combs and cutlery (Fig. 10), and many other simple measures, preserve independence. More sophisticated examples include the raised toilet seat and the tipping table for kettles. Many of these devices are available at local shops, but whenever possible the occupational therapists should be asked to help assess and advise patients.

Major alterations to the patient's home or environment may be necessary to allow the severely disabled to go on living independently. It is then essential to involve the OTs and social services. Common alterations include stair lifts and ramps. The 'Possum' system and other electronic devices may be used to allow people with very little movement to continue to carry out complex tasks at home.

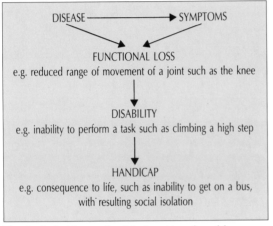

Fig. 8 *Arthritis can lead to functional problems, disability and handicap.*

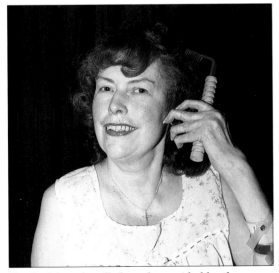

Fig. 9 *A long-handled comb provided by the occupational therapist helps this patient with rheumatoid arthritis and severe elbow, shoulder and wrist involvement to comb her hair.*

Example

Sandra is 67. She has severe rheumatoid arthritis. While her husband Frank was still alive she managed well enough; he helped her dress and get up and down the stairs, and he did many of the household chores. Frank had a sudden, fatal coronary two years ago, leaving Sandra on her own. She quickly realized that she couldn't manage. For a while friends and neighbours helped out, but Sandra knew that she could not go on that way. Her GP called in the domiciliary OT and the social services, and they all got together to help Sandra sort things out. Problems with dressing, washing and cooking were easily sorted out with the help of a dressing stick and some other simple aids, as well as some reorganization of the kitchen and bathroom. The stairs were a bigger problem. Sandra had to live downstairs for a while, and use a commode. But she recently had a stair lift put in, and she is now managing nearly as well as she was before Frank died.

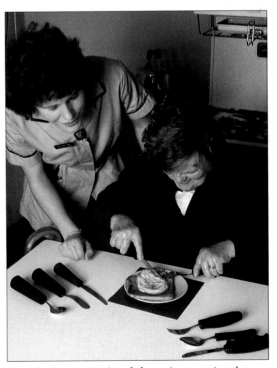

Fig. 10 *An occupational therapist assessing the use of various cutlery grips to aid eating. Restricted finger flexion from rheumatoid arthritis means that the patient can only grasp large diameter handles.*

WALKING AIDS

The Problem

- Musculoskeletal problems often cause pain and difficulty with standing and walking.
- Walking difficulties are often due to mechanical factors, such as joint deformity or instability, as well as accompanying muscle weakness. They may not be totally correctable.
- Pain on walking may be due to normal loading of abnormal joints, or to abnormal loading resulting from altered lower-limb biomechanics.
- Abnormal joints may be vulnerable to further damage if exposed to excessive loading.

Why Intervene?

- To reduce pain on walking.
- To increase mobility, walking range, and independence.
- To correct abnormal loading of joints.
- To protect abnormal joints from excessive loading.

What is There?

Shoes: good shoes should avoid excessive, localized pressure on the foot and allow normal weight distribution. The abnormal shape of the arthritic foot often requires wide-fitting, deep shoes, and Velcro fastenings across the front may help the patient who also has an arthritic hand (Fig. 11). Modifications to shoes can relieve pressure on painful areas, support falling arches, and compensate for angulation deformities of the lower limb. The importance of footwear cannot be overstressed, and it is worth finding out what local cobblers and shops have available (for example, wide-fitting shoes), as well as knowing what local hospital fitters and chiropodists can do.
Sticks: a walking stick is one of the simplest, most important and most ill-used aids. A good stick needs to be the right length, have a non-slip ferrule and an appropriate handle (Fig. 12). Correct use, on the opposite side to the painful hip or knee, or on the same side if there is instability, reduces loading and pain, and can make a big difference to confidence, stability and mobility.
Crutches and frames: these can be used to achieve

greater reduction of loading, with less stress on the upper limbs and greater security than can be provided by sticks.

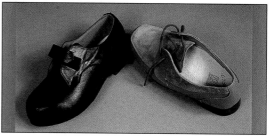

Fig. 11 *Two types of shoe available to arthritis sufferers. Note the deep fitting, wide shoe which can accommodate deformed feet, and easy-to-use Velcro fastenings.*

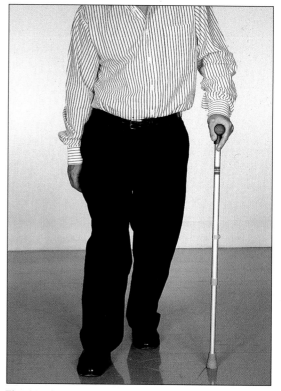

Fig. 12 *Correct use of a walking stick can make an enormous difference to someone with hip or knee disease. For pain relief the stick, which should reach the height of the femoral greater trochanter, should be held in the opposite hand.*

Example

John is a 63-year-old man who developed osteo-arthritis of the right hip in his early fifties. In his mid-fifties he noticed that he was in considerable pain on walking and could not manage more than half a mile without stopping. He started using a stick, and found that it dramatically reduced pain on walking. This helped keep him going for a number of years. However, at the age of 61 the hip got a lot worse over a period of a few months. John was in great pain and very handicapped. He had a success-ful hip replacement last year, but was left with some inequality in leg length. This has been corrected by a heel raise to his left shoe; the result has been much less backache, due to reduced stress on the spine on walking.

DRUG TREATMENT

The Problem

- There is no known cure for the major rheumatic disorders, such as rheumatoid arthritis and osteo-arthritis. Drug therapy is therefore used to alleviate the major symptoms of pain or inflammation resulting from these disorders.
- In certain circumstances, for example active rheumatoid arthritis, drugs are also used in an attempt to switch off the underlying disease process and provide additional suppression of symptoms.
- Pharmacological management of rheumatic dis-orders requires careful consideration of the balance between the risks and benefits of any agent (Fig. 13).

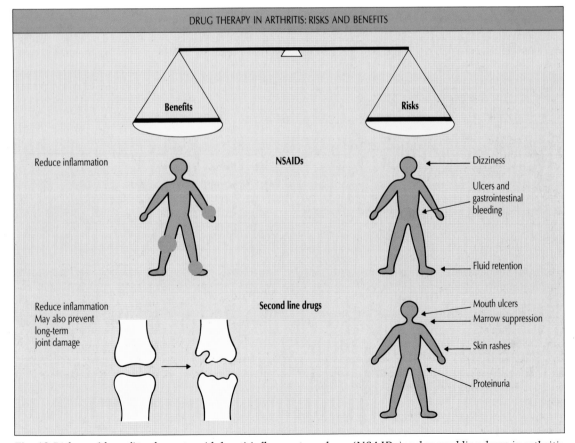

Fig. 13 *Risks and benefits of nonsteroidal anti-inflammatory drugs (NSAIDs) and second line drugs in arthritis.*

Why Intervene?

- Mechanical pain, common in osteoarthritis, can often be controlled with analgesic drugs.
- Pain, swelling and stiffness are major features of inflammatory joint disorders such as rheumatoid arthritis. These symptoms and signs are best treated with nonsteroidal anti-inflammatory drugs. If severe symptoms persist, inflammation may be reduced by the addition of 'second line' drugs (Fig. 14). These agents require close monitoring for adverse effects (Fig. 15).

SECOND LINE DRUGS IN RHEUMATOID ARTHRITIS	
Gold	Azothiaprine
Penicillamine	Methotrexate
Hydroxychloroquine	Auranofin
Sulphalasalazine	

Fig. 14 *Second line drugs in rheumatoid arthritis.*

What is There?

Analgesics: the best ones to use in the setting of chronic musculoskeletal pain are those relatively free of central nervous system and gut side-effects, such as paracetamol alone or with dextropropoxyphene.

Analgesics are particularly useful where structural changes not amenable to mechanical aids or surgery are a major cause of symptoms, and they are the drug treatment of choice in osteoarthritis.

- The relationship between pain and the patient's environment and psychological state are relevant in determining response to analgesic therapy.
- They should be taken regularly, at times and in doses which relate to symptoms.

Nonsteroidal anti-inflammatory drugs (NSAIDs): this group comprises a large number of agents (Fig. 16) which are thought to act by inhibition of enzymes that produce potent inflammatory molecules (prostaglandins).

The major adverse effect of NSAIDs is gastrointestinal irritation, particularly mucosal ulceration and haemorrhage. Several attempts have been made to overcome gastric irritability, including enteric coating, rectal administration, formulation of prodrugs (inactive agents converted to the active form at a site distant from the stomach) and concomitant administration of anti-ulcer drugs. These measures have succeeded in reducing but not abolishing the risk of gastrointestinal adverse effects.

- Make a small selection and get to know them well.
- Prescribe one NSAID at a time.
- Prescribe for a limited period (e.g. 3 weeks) but in an adequate dose, before deciding on therapeutic success or failure.
- Relate timing to symptoms. Slow-release, long half-life preparations at night may relieve morning symptoms.
- Be wary of their use in the elderly, as side-effects are more frequent and more serious.

Example

Edith is a 55-year-old housewife who gave a six-month history of pain, swelling and morning stiffness in her metacarpophalangeal joints, knees and feet. Serological indices (plasma viscosity and C-reactive protein) were markedly elevated, she was positive for rheumatoid factor and radiographs revealed soft-tissue swelling but no erosions in the small joints of her hands and feet. She had clearly developed rheumatoid arthritis.

Edith tried taking aspirin when her joints felt particularly bad, but she didn't notice any marked improvement from this. Many of her symptoms stemmed from active joint inflammation, and she was prescribed an adequate dose of a nonsteroidal anti-inflammatory regularly. On this regimen, her arthritis settled and remained quiescent for four months. It then flared up again, this time additionally affecting the elbows, shoulders and ankles. There was little improvement with bed-rest and three nonsteroidal anti-inflammatories had been tried, with little effect. Radiographs of her feet showed evidence of a few erosions in the metatarsophalangeal joints.

Her disease had remained active and was clearly beginning to induce structural joint damage. She was then referred to a rheumatologist and gold injections were commenced, with monthly monitoring of her full blood count and urine protein. Over a six-month period, her disease has gradually become less active, and her functional ability has been improving.

HOW TO MONITOR SECOND LINE DRUGS IN RHEUMATOID ARTHRITIS*				
Monthly tests required:				

	FBC	Platelets	LFTs	Urine
Gold	●	●		●
Penicillamine	●	●		●
Sulphasalazine	●	●		
Azothiaprine	●	●		
Methotrexate	●	●	●	
Auranofin	●	●		●
Hydroxychloroquine	●	●		

FBC   = Full blood count
Platelets = Platelet count
LFTs   = Liver function tests
              (transaminases, alkaline phosphatase)
Urine   = Dipstick test for proteinuria

Action

FBC: Stop drug if *total* white cell count $<3.5 \times 10^9/l$
              or if granulocyte count $<2.0 \times 10^9/l$

Platelets: Stop drug if patient count $<100 \times 10^9/l$ (ensure that
              the thrombocytopenia is not artefactual, i.e. due to
              platelet clumping — repeat test if in doubt)

LFTs: Stop the drug (methotrexate) if the rise in transamin-
              ases or alkaline phosphatase exceeds three times the
              normal range (a small rise in these parameters is usual)

Urine: If dipstick testing reveals more than 1+ proteinuria,
              which is confirmed on repeat testing one week later,
              perform a 24-hour urine collection to measure total
              protein excretion. If this exceeds 1g per 24 hours
              stop the drug. Recheck 24-hour protein excretion at
              monthly intervals — the patient may be rechallenged
              if the proteinuria resolves

FOR FURTHER ADVICE CONTACT YOUR RHEUMATOLOGY UNIT FIRST.

*As practiced in the Rheumatology Unit, Bristol Royal Infirmary, at the time of going to press.

Fig. 15 *Monitoring of second-line drug therapy.*

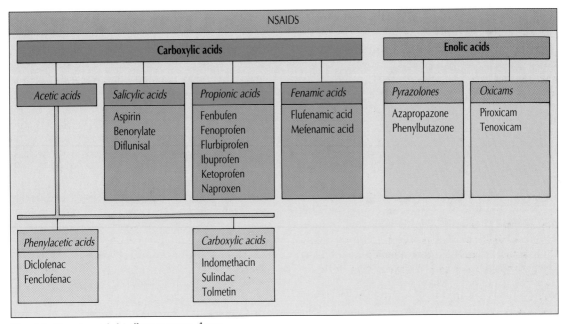

Fig. 16 *Nonsteroidal inflammatory drugs.*

LOCAL INJECTION TREATMENT

The Problem

- Soft-tissue disorders, such as tendonitis and inflammation at tendonous or ligamentous insertions, often resolve slowly.
- Synovitis affecting tendon sheaths or bursae is often well-localized and may not respond to systemic therapy.
- Many generalized rheumatic disorders are characterized by exacerbations in one joint from time to time.

Why Intervene?

- There is a possibility of accelerated and effective mobilization when local injection is used in combination with physiotherapy.
- A rapid reduction in synovitis, with relief of pain and stiffness, can be achieved within 12–48 hours.
- The response to systemic treatment (nonsteroidal anti-inflammatory or second line drug) in inflammatory arthritides is often slow.

What is There?

Steroids are the drugs most commonly given in local injections.

Steroid injections should be avoided if the diagnosis is not definitely known. The speed of onset and duration of response varies with the steroid type used, the underlying condition and the site injected.

When using injections for localized soft-tissue disorders:

- The precise point of greatest tenderness should be infiltrated.
- Use of local anaesthetic confirms precise siting of the injection. Local anaesthetic should be avoided when injections are given close to nerves (carpal tunnel syndrome or the elbow).
- Tell the patient to avoid overuse for 72 hours after injection.
- Do not inject into tendons as these may rupture.

When injecting joints, certain precautions should always be observed:

- Do not inject in the presence of local or systemic infection.
- Use aseptic technique.
- Be sure the needle is in the synovial space — confirmed by aspirating fluid or ease of injection.
- Do not inject if aspirated fluid is heavily blood-stained.
- Always send aspirated fluid for culture.

Non-weightbearing joints show more prolonged improvement than weightbearing joints. Major complications such as infection are extremely rare. Good technique is important if tendon rupture and muscle atrophy are to be avoided.

Example

Herbert, a 50-year-old roofer, presented with a two-week history of pain and stiffness of his right shoulder. The symptoms commenced after he had to perform a week of unusually strenuous heavy lifting in his workplace. On examination there was painful limited active abduction of his right glenohumeral joint to 90°, but passive abduction was possible to 140°.

The history and physical findings were strongly suggestive of a rotator cuff tendonitis. Forty milligrams of a long-acting steroid preparation (steroids such as triamcinolone are suitable) was infiltrated along the track of the supraspinatus tendon, using a 21 gauge needle and a lateral approach. Care was taken not to inject directly into the joint. One millilitre of 1% lignocaine had been mixed in with the steroid, and within a few minutes pain-free active abduction was possible, demonstrating that the injection had reached the appropriate site. Herbert was able to return to his work after a two-week period of rest followed by shoulder exercises (see p.5.5).

SURGERY

The Problem

- Arthritis can destroy joints and periarticular tissues.
- Destroyed joints may be painful, unstable or immobile (or have any combination of these three features of 'joint failure').
- Alterations in joint anatomy and periarticular tissues can cause secondary pressure on vital structures, particularly the spinal cord, nerve roots or peripheral nerves.
- Destroyed joints rarely heal, although patients can adapt to the consequent problems, pain may settle, and damaged joints sometimes fuse spontaneously.

Why Intervene?

- Surgery is one of the most effective means of relieving pain and improving function in severe arthritis.
- Immediate surgery may be necessary to prevent progressive neurological damage in severe disc disease and other local nerve-pressure problems.
- The difficult decision in other cases is often *when* to intervene, and *what* to do, rather than *why*.
- Severe pain (especially night pain) in spite of other more conservative measures, with or without severe disability (less than 15 minutes standing or walking time, for example), are the usual indications for surgery.
- In arthritic patients with multiple problems, the decision to operate should ideally be taken by the patient after joint consultation with a surgeon and physician, aided by the paramedical team who can assess the likely functional outcome.
- Before referring patients for surgery, it is important to find out what local, combined services are available.

What is There?

Joint replacement is increasingly successful for an enlarging number of joints. Hip and knee replacements remain the most important.

Osteotomy (realignment of bones) is sometimes valuable in knee osteoarthritis, and in certain foot deformities (for example hallux valgus).

Arthrodesis (joint fusion) is rarely necessary except for the painful, unstable rheumatoid wrist, ankle or thumb interphalangeal joint, or as a salvage procedure (Fig. 17).

Synovectomy (removal of synovium) is of limited value, and is now usually performed by injection of radiocolloids rather than by surgery (Fig. 17).

Soft tissue reconstructive surgery is very important, particularly in the maintenance and improvement of hand function. Tendon reconstruction (e.g. for dropped fingers due to rupture of extensor tendons) and release of soft tissue contractures are examples (Fig. 17).

Decompression operations may be necessary for severe carpal tunnel syndrome, for disc disease with root or cord compression, and for spinal stenosis or rheumatoid cervical spine disease with cord involvement (Fig. 17).

Example

Alice is a 53-year-old lady with severe rheumatoid arthritis, which began at the age of 28. She has had a variety of treatments, including three operations.

Her feet were troublesome from the beginning. She experienced a lot of pain under the toes on walking. For a while this seemed to be controlled by adapting her shoes, but it worsened until she felt she was walking on stones. In addition, her toes became cocked-up, rubbing on the inside of the shoe. A 'Fowler's' operation was carried out, removing the ends of the metatarsals. Alice was delighted with the result, and her feet have been largely pain free ever since.

Her right knee became painful a few years later. It wasn't too troublesome to begin with but it suddenly worsened. When she reported severe night pain and a walking time of less than 10 minutes she was referred to a combined orthopaedic and rheumatology clinic. The rheumatologists checked her general health and agreed with the surgical recommendation. A knee prosthesis was inserted, with an excellent result.

Alice's most recent operation was on her right hand. Her wrist had been playing up, making gripping things awkward. One morning she woke up to find that she couldn't straighten out her ring and little finger. After another consultation in the combined clinic, and an assessment of hand function by the occupational (remedial) therapist, she agreed to surgery. The ulnar styloid was removed, and the damaged wrist arthrodesed. The ruptured extensor tendons were reconstructed. After an extended period of intensive post-operative physiotherapy, a reasonable return of function was obtained, and the wrist is now pain free.

FOUR TYPES OF SURGICAL PROCEDURE

1. **Decompression** operations are sometimes necessary to relieve pressure on vital structures
Example: carpal tunnel syndrome

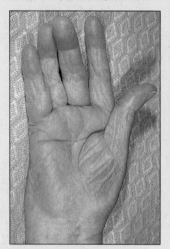 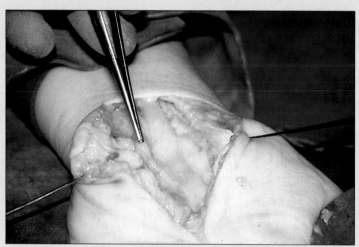

2. **Synovectomy** is sometimes useful to relieve symptoms, and prophylacticlly to prevent damage to tendons and ligaments
Example: dorsal synovectomy of the wrist

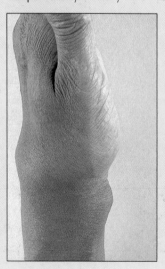 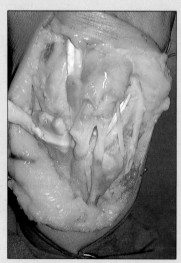 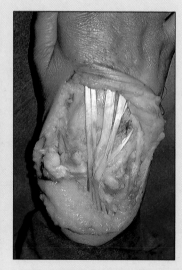

3. **Reconstructive surgery** can return function after ligament or tendon rupture
Example: flexor tendon sheath

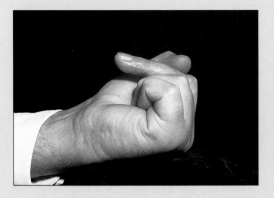
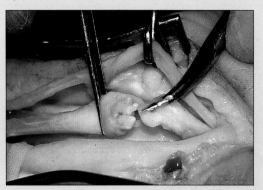

4. **Arthroplasty** can be carried out to relieve pain and improve function of badly damaged joints
Example: MCP joint replacement

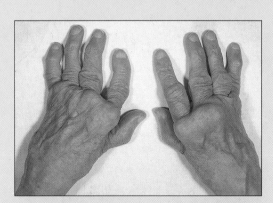
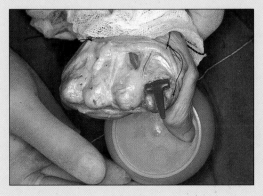
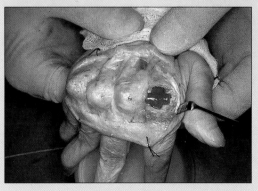

Fig. 17 *Four types of surgical procedure.*

INDEX